LOW SODIUM

RECIPES

A Low Sodium Cookbook for Eating Healthy

(Low Sodium, Low Phosphorus Healthy Recipes to Avoid
Dialysis and Stay Healthy)

Jack Overman

Published by Alex Howard

© **Jack Overman**

All Rights Reserved

Low Sodium Recipes: A Low Sodium Cookbook for Eating Healthy (Low Sodium, Low Phosphorus Healthy Recipes to Avoid Dialysis and Stay Healthy)

ISBN 978-1-990169-76-2

Legal & Disclaimer

The information contained in this book is not designed to replace or take the place of any form of medicine or professional medical advice. The information in this book has been provided for educational and entertainment purposes only.

Table of contents

Part 1

Introduction

If you are reading this book, you or someone you know probably suffers from kidney-related ailments. And you are not alone; there are millions of people around the world who suffer from kidney diseases. This book is meant for people who want to make better health choices for improving kidney health.

A person with kidney disease has specific needs that have to be met. Their diet has to comprise of very low amounts of sodium, potassium, and phosphorus. Just the fact that salt has to be reduced can mean your food tastes very different. Making these food choices can be quite tough for most people. They usually feel as though the taste or flavor has been taken away from their food. However, this does not have to be true.

This cookbook has been put together in a way that you can follow a healthy renal friendly diet while still enjoying your food. You will first be learning a little more about the renal diet and foods that you should or should not eat. Then you can get started with trying out the numerous kidney-friendly recipes in the book. You will soon see that being healthy does not have to mean making a compromise on delicious food. There are enough recipes here for you to enjoy a versatile meal plan for a long time.

Chapter 1: What is the Renal Diet and How Does it Help You?

A renal diet comprises of foods that are good for the kidney. People who are suffering from any kidney-related diseases or conditions would benefit from following this diet. An ailing kidney can affect your overall health and life in many ways. This is why we have put together this renal diet cookbook to help you or anyone who needs it. This renal diet will not cure your disease or cause any drastic changes in your health in a week. However, these nutritional choices will make a difference in the long term and prevent further damage to your kidney. It can also greatly help in reducing the severity of your condition.

A good renal diet will help in controlling the amount of sodium, potassium, phosphorus, and protein that you consume. You will learn to avoid foods that harm your kidney and contain too much of these ingredients. The diet will also help in reducing the amount of waste produced by your body. This is important so that the workload of your kidneys is reduced, and kidney function can be preserved for longer. Chronic kidney disease can be a very tricky condition to deal with, and you have to take as many steps as possible to take care of your kidney. The renal diet is known to help in slowing the progress of kidney disease. It may help in delaying the need for dialysis or any renal failure for quite some time. On the other hand, following your usual unhealthy diet can accelerate the rate at which your kidney function decays. It may seem like a lot of work to follow this type of diet, but this is why we have put together this book for you. It will take a little time to get used to it, but you will be able to succeed in the long term. Following a renal diet will not mean eating bland food for the rest of your life. Instead, this cookbook will help you be more imaginative with your meals and enjoy delicious food.

The following tips will help you follow a healthy renal diet.

Tips for Renal Diet

Understand more about kidney disease. The more well informed you are, the better you will be able to deal with your condition. Don't just depend on a doctor telling you what to do. Ask questions, and try to understand why you have to make changes in your diet and lifestyle. This will help you a lot in the long term, and you will be able to live more empowered despite your disease.

Control your consumption of the following:

- Sodium
- Potassium
- Protein
- Fats
- Phosphorus
- Carbohydrates
- Vitamins

- Minerals
- Fluids

Don't add salt to your food while cooking or eating.

Be more conscious of the labels on any food you buy. Check the ingredient list. Anything with more than 300mg of sodium per serving should be avoided.

Renal Friendly Foods
- Vegetables like red bell peppers, cabbage, radish, turnips, cauliflower, garlic, onions,
- Fruits like apples, cranberries, pineapple, blueberries, raspberries, strawberries, cherries, and red grapes.
- Eggs, specifically egg whites, are better.
- Fish like Sea Bass.
- Olive oil.
- Fresh chicken, skinless.
- Greens like Arugula that is low in potassium.
- Shitake mushrooms.
- Macadamia Nuts.

Foods to Avoid:
- Soft drinks.
- Canned foods.
- Dried beans.
- Fruits like Avocados, Bananas, Oranges, and Apricots.
- Whole wheat bread.
- Brown rice.
- Dairy products.
- Pickles.

- Beer.
- Olives.
- Vegetables like Tomatoes, Pumpkin, Winter Squash, Potatoes, and Sweet potatoes.
- Any pre-made meals or packaged food.
- Greens like Spinach, Beet Greens, Kale, and Swiss chard.
- Dried fruits like raisins, prunes and dates.
- Snacks like chips, crackers, or pretzels.

Chapter 2: Juices and Drinks

Blueberry Blast Smoothie

Number of servings: 2

Nutritional values per serving:

Calories – 108, Fat – 0 g, Carbohydrate – 18 g, Fiber – 1.2 g, Protein – 9 g, Sodium – 27 mg, Potassium – 183 mg, Phosphorous – 42 mg, Calcium – 57 mg

Ingredients:
- ½ cup frozen blueberries
- 3 tablespoons protein powder (preferably egg white or whey protein powder)
- 7 ounces apple juice, unsweetened
- 4 packets Splenda or to taste
- 4 ice cubes

Directions:
1. Gather all the ingredients and add into a blender.
2. Blend for 30 – 40 seconds or until smooth.
3. Pour into 2 glasses and serve.

Fruity Smoothie

Number of servings: 1

Nutritional values per serving:

Calories – 186, Fat – 2 g, Carbohydrate – 19 g, Fiber – 1.1 g, Protein – 23 g, Sodium – 62 mg, Potassium – 282 mg, Phosphorous – 118 mg, Calcium – 160 mg

Ingredients:

- 4 ounces fruit cocktail, with its juice
- ½ cup cold water
- 1 scoop vanilla whey protein powder
- ½ cup crushed ice

Directions:

1. Gather all the ingredients and add into a blender.
2. Blend for 30 – 40 seconds or until smooth.
3. Pour into a tall glass and serve.

Pineapple Protein Smoothie

Number of servings: 2

Nutritional values per serving:

Calories – 268, Fat – 4 g, Carbohydrate – 40 g, Fiber – 1.4 g, Protein – 18 g, Sodium 93 mg, Potassium – 237 mg, Phosphorous – 160 mg, Calcium – 160 mg

Ingredients:

- 1 ½ cups pineapple sherbet or sorbet
- 1 cup water
- 2 scoops vanilla whey protein powder
- Ice cubes, as required (optional)

Directions:

1. Gather all the ingredients and add into a blender.
2. Blend for 30 – 40 seconds or until smooth.
3. Pour into 2 glasses and serve.

Easy No Milk Shake

Number of servings: 2

Nutritional values per serving:

Calories – 203, Fat – NA, Carbohydrate – NA, Fiber – NA, Protein – 19 g, Sodium – 195 mg, Potassium – 52 mg, Phosphorous – 1 mg, Calcium – NA

Ingredients:

- 2 cups pasteurized liquid egg product
- ½ teaspoon almond extract or vanilla extract or 1 tablespoon lemon juice
- 1 cup frozen non-dairy whipped topping
- 1 cup berries
- 1 apple, cored, chopped
- 3-4 tablespoons plain peanut butter, unsalted (optional)

Directions:

1. Gather all the ingredients and add into a blender.
2. Blend for 30 – 40 seconds or until smooth.
3. Pour into 2 glasses and serve.

Very Berry Tofu Smoothie

Number of servings: 2

Nutritional values per serving:

Calories – 125, Fat – 1.8 g, Carbohydrate – 22 g, Fiber – 6 g, Protein – 6 g, Sodium – 42 mg, Potassium – 339 mg, Phosphorous – 100 mg, Calcium – 44 mg

Ingredients:

- 1 cup blueberries
- ½ pound fresh strawberries, chopped
- ¼ teaspoon ground ginger
- 1/8 teaspoon rum extract
- ½ teaspoon lemon juice
- 4.5 ounces silken tofu
- A pinch red pepper flakes
- ½ tablespoon honey
- Ice cubes, as required

Directions:

1. Gather all the ingredients and add into a blender.
2. Blend for 30 – 40 seconds or until smooth.
3. Pour into 2 glasses and serve.

Peach High-Protein Fruit Smoothie

Number of servings: 2

Nutritional values per serving:

Calories – 132, Fat – 0 g, Carbohydrate – 24 g, Fiber – 1.9 g, Protein – 10 g, Sodium – 154 mg, Potassium – 353 mg, Phosphorous – 36 mg, Calcium – 9 mg

Ingredients:

- 4 tablespoons Just Whites (powdered egg whites)
- 2 tablespoons sugar
- 1 cup ice
- 1 ½ cups fresh peaches

Directions:

1. Gather all the ingredients and add peaches into a blender.
2. Blend for 30 – 40 seconds or until smooth.
3. Add rest of the ingredients and blend until smooth.
4. Pour into 2 glasses and serve.

Strawberry High-Protein Fruit Smoothie

Number of servings: 2

Nutritional values per serving:

Calories – 156, Fat – 0 g, Carbohydrate – 25 g, Fiber – 2.5 g, Protein – 14 g, Sodium – 215 mg, Potassium – 400 mg, Phosphorous – 49 mg, Calcium – 29 mg

Ingredients:

- 1 ½ cups chopped, fresh strawberries
- 1 cup ice cubes
- 1 cup liquid pasteurized egg whites
- 2 tablespoons sugar

Directions:

1. Gather all the ingredients and add strawberries into a blender.
2. Blend for 30 – 40 seconds or until smooth.
3. Add rest of the ingredients and blend until smooth.
4. Pour into 2 glasses and serve.

Mixed Berry Protein Smoothie

Number of servings: 1

Nutritional values per serving:

Calories – 104, Fat – 4 g, Carbohydrate – 11 g, Fiber – 2.4 g, Protein – 6 g, Sodium – 15 mg, Potassium – 141 mg, Phosphorous – 49 mg, Calcium – 69 mg

Ingredients:

- ½ cup frozen mixed berries
- ½ teaspoon Crystal Light liquid flavor enhancer drops, blueberry raspberry flavor
- 1 scoop whey protein powder
- 2 ounces chilled water
- 1 ice cube
- ¼ cup whipped cream topping

Directions:

1. Gather all the ingredients and add berries, water, liquid flavor enhancer drops, and ice cube into a blender.
2. Blend for 30 – 40 seconds or until slush-like inconsistency.
3. Add whipped topping and protein powder and blend until well combined.
4. Pour into a tall glass and serve.

Green Juice

Number of servings: 1

Nutritional values per serving:

Calories – 130, Fat – 1 g, Carbohydrate – 31 g, Fiber – 0 g, Protein – 1 g, Sodium – 4 mg, Potassium – 366 mg, Phosphorous – 46 mg, Calcium – 33 mg

Ingredients:

- 1 medium green apple, cored, sliced
- ¼ cup chopped fresh pineapple
- 1 tablespoon lemon juice
- 1 small cucumber, chopped

Directions:

1. Juice together all the fruits and cucumber in a juicer.
2. Pour into a glass. Stir in lemon juice and serve.

Fabulous Hot Cocoa

Number of servings: 2

Nutritional values per serving:

Calories – 72, Fat – 3 g, Carbohydrate – 13 g, Fiber – 1.8 g, Protein – 1 g, Sodium – 10 mg, Potassium – 100 mg, Phosphorous – 49 mg, Calcium – 26 mg

Ingredients:

- 2 cups boiling water
- 4 teaspoons granulated sugar
- 6 tablespoons whipped dessert topping
- 2 tablespoons cocoa powder, unsweetened
- 4 tablespoons cold water

Directions:

1. Add cocoa powder, sugar, and cold water into a bowl and stir until well combined.
2. Divide into 2 cups.
3. Pour a cup of hot water into each cup. Stir until sugar dissolves completely.
4. Divide the dessert topping among the cups and serve.

Chapter Three: Breakfast Recipes

Acai Berry Smoothie Bowl

Number of servings: 1

Nutritional values per serving:

Calories – 192, Fat – 4 g, Carbohydrate – 28 g, Fiber – 7.2 g, Protein – 11 g, Sodium – 82 mg, Potassium – 349 mg, Phosphorous – 140 mg, Calcium – 298 mg

Ingredients:

For smoothie bowl:

- ½ packet frozen acai, unsweetened
- 6 tablespoons plain 2 % low-fat Greek yogurt
- ¼ cup rice milk, unsweetened
- ½ cup frozen mixed berries, unsweetened
- ½ teaspoon chia seeds

For topping:

- 1 tablespoon blueberries
- 1 tablespoon raspberries
- 1/8 fresh pear, chopped

Directions:

1. Break the frozen acai into smaller pieces and add into a blender.
2. Add rest of the ingredients for smoothie bowl into the blender and blend until creamy.
3. Pour into a bowl.

4. Scatter blueberries, raspberries, and pear on top and serve.

Apple Cinnamon Maple Granola

Number of servings: 8

Nutritional values per serving: ½ cup without milk

Calories – 162, Fat – 6 g, Carbohydrate – 25 g, Fiber – 2.6 g, Protein – 2 g, Sodium – 3 mg, Potassium – 107 mg, Phosphorous – 70 mg, Calcium – 18 mg

Ingredients:

- 1 ½ cups puffed rice cereal
- 1.7 ounces baked apple chips
- 1 ½ cups old fashioned oats
- ¼ cup dried, sweetened cranberries
- ½ teaspoon ground nutmeg
- 2 tablespoons 100% pure maple syrup
- ¼ cup unsweetened applesauce
- ¾ teaspoon ground cinnamon
- 2 tablespoons melted coconut oil
- ¾ teaspoon vanilla extract

Directions:

1. Place a sheet of parchment paper on a large baking sheet.
2. Add all the dry ingredients into a bowl and toss well.
3. Add all the wet ingredients into another bowl and whisk well. Drizzle over the dry ingredients and toss until well coated.
4. Spread onto the prepared baking sheet.

5.   Bake in a preheated oven at 275° F for about 50 – 60 minutes. Stir a couple of times while baking.

6.   Cool completely. Transfer into an airtight container and store at room temperature. It can last for a week.

7. To serve: Place ½ cup granola in a bowl. Pour some rice milk or almond milk and serve.

Baked Egg Cups

Number of servings: 6

Nutritional values per serving:

Calories – 80, Fat – 5 g, Carbohydrate – 1 g, Fiber – 0.1 g, Protein – 7 g, Sodium – 78 mg, Potassium – 92 mg, Phosphorous – 101 mg, Calcium – 28 mg

Ingredients:

- 3 slices low-sodium bacon, cooked crisp, crumbled
- 3 tablespoons chopped mushrooms
- 3 tablespoons chopped onions
- 3 tablespoons chopped bell pepper
- 1/8 teaspoon pepper
- 6 large eggs

Directions:

1. Take a 6 counts muffin pan and line it disposable muffin liners.
2. Add bacon and vegetables into a bowl and toss well.
3. Divide into the muffin cups.

4. Add eggs and pepper into another bowl and whisk well. Divide into the muffin cups.
5. Bake in a preheated oven at 350° F for about 20-30 minutes or until the eggs are set well.
6. Remove the muffin pan from the oven and let it cool for a couple of minutes. Loosen the edges of the muffins with a knife and remove the muffins.
7. Serve immediately.

Egg White French Toast

Number of servings: 2

Nutritional values per serving:

Calories – 200, Fat – 5 g, Carbohydrate – 24 g, Fiber – 0.7 g, Protein – 15 g, Sodium – 415 mg, Potassium – 235 mg, Phosphorous – 54 mg, Calcium – 50 mg

Ingredients:

- 2 slices bread
- 1 cup egg whites
- 2 teaspoons unsalted butter, softened
- 4 tablespoons sugar-free syrup

Directions:

1. Apply butter over the bread slices. Chop into 1-inch cubes and place in a microwave-safe bowl.
2. Whisk egg whites and pour over the bread.
3. Drizzle syrup all over the whites.
4. Microwave on high for 60 to 70 seconds. Slightly lift the egg whites.
5. Cook for 40-60 seconds until eggs are set.
6. Serve hot.

Fluffy Homemade Buttermilk Pancakes

Number of servings: 4 pancakes of 4 inches and one of 2 inches

Nutritional values per serving: 1 pancake without berries

Calories – 217, Fat – 9 g, Carbohydrate – 27 g, Fiber – 1 g, Protein – 6 g, Sodium – 330 mg, Potassium – 182 mg, Phosphorous – 100 mg, Calcium – 74 mg

Ingredients:

For dry ingredients:

- 1 cup all-purpose flour
- ¾ teaspoon baking soda
- 1 cup low-fat buttermilk
- 2 ½ tablespoons canola oil, divided
- ½ teaspoon cream of tartar
- 1 tablespoon sugar
- 1 large egg

Directions:

1. Add all the dry ingredients into a mixing bowl.
2. Add all the wet ingredients (set aside ½ tablespoon of the oil) into another bowl and whisk well.
3. Pour the wet ingredients into the bowl of dry ingredients and whisk well.
4. Place a skillet over medium heat. Brush with some of the remaining oil. When the pan is heated, pour 1/3 cup of the batter on the skillet. Spread the pancakes with the back of a spoon to about 4 inches

in diameter. If your pan is large, you can make 2 pancakes at a time.

5. In a while, bubbles will appear on the pancakes. Cook until the underside is golden brown. Flip sides and cook the other side until golden brown.
6. Remove onto a plate.
7. Repeat steps 4 – 6 and make the remaining pancakes.
8. Serve with fresh berries if desired.

Blueberry Muffins

Number of servings: 6

Nutritional values per serving: 1 muffin

Calories – 275, Fat – 9 g, Carbohydrate – 44 g, Fiber – 1.3 g, Protein – 5 g, Sodium – 210 mg, Potassium – 121 mg, Phosphorous – 100 mg, Calcium – 108 mg

Ingredients:

- ¼ cup unsalted butter or margarine
- 1 egg
- 1 cup all-purpose flour
- ¼ teaspoon salt
- 10 tablespoons + 1 teaspoon sugar
- 1 cup 1% milk
- 1 teaspoon baking powder
- 1 ¼ cup fresh blueberries

Directions:

1. Add butter and sugar (except 1 teaspoon sugar) into a mixing bowl and beat with an electric hand mixer on low speed until smooth and creamy.
2. Beat in the egg.
3. Add dry ingredients into another bowl and stir. Add into the bowl of butter mixture, a little at a time alternating with a little milk each time.
4. Add ¼ cup blueberries into a bowl and mash them. Add into the batter and mix using your hands.
5. Add the rest of the blueberries and mix using your hands.

6. Grease a 6-count muffin cup with cooking spray.
7. Divide the batter among the muffin cups. Sprinkle 1-teaspoon sugar on top of the batter in the muffin cups.
8. Bake in a preheated oven at 375° F for about 25 – 30 minutes.
9. Remove the muffins from the oven and cool for 35 – 40 minutes and serve.

Spicy Tofu Scramble

Number of servings: 4

Nutritional values per serving:

Calories – 213, Fat – 13 g, Carbohydrate – 10 g, Fiber – 2 g, Protein – 18 g, Sodium – 24 mg, Potassium – 242 mg, Phosphorous – 467 mg, Calcium – 274 mg

Ingredients:

- 2 teaspoons olive oil
- ½ cup chopped green bell pepper
- ½ cup chopped red bell pepper
- 2 cups drained, crumbled firm tofu (with less than 10% calcium)
- ½ teaspoon garlic powder
- ¼ teaspoon ground turmeric
- 2 teaspoons onion powder
- 2 cloves garlic, minced

Directions:

1. Place a nonstick pan over medium heat. Add oil. When the oil is heated, add garlic and bell peppers and sauté for 2-3 minutes.
2. Add rest of the ingredients and mix well. Cook until most of the tofu is light golden brown in color. Stir occasionally.
3. Serve hot.

Loaded Veggie Eggs

Number of servings: 1

Nutritional values per serving:

Calories – 240, Fat – 16.6 g, Carbohydrate – 7.8 g, Fiber – 2.7 g, Protein – 15.3 g, Sodium – 195 mg, Potassium – 602 mg, Phosphorous – 253 mg, Calcium – NA

Ingredients:

- 2 whole eggs
- 1 ½ cups fresh spinach
- 2 tablespoons chopped bell pepper
- ½ cup chopped cauliflower
- 2 small cloves garlic, minced
- 2 tablespoons chopped onion
- ½ tablespoon coconut oil or avocado oil
- Pepper to taste
- A handful fresh parsley, chopped, to garnish

Directions:

1. Add eggs and pepper into a bowl and beat until frothy.
2. Place a skillet over medium heat. Add oil. When the oil is heated, add onion and bell pepper and cook until tender.
3. Add garlic and stir for a few seconds until aromatic.
4. Stir in the cauliflower and spinach. Lower the heat to medium-low. Cover and cook for 3-4 minutes.
5. Stir in the eggs. Stir frequently until eggs are set.

6. Garnish with parsley and serve. If you want to reduce potassium further, replace 2 whole eggs with 4 whites.

Spinach Ricotta Frittata

Number of servings: 3

Nutritional values per serving:

Calories – 220, Fat – 15 g, Carbohydrate – 6 g, Fiber – 7 g, Protein – 16 g, Sodium – 174 mg, Potassium – 255 mg, Phosphorous – 203 mg, Calcium – NA

Ingredients:

- 5 omega 3 eggs
- ½ tablespoon fresh chopped herbs
- 1 small onion, chopped
- 1 ½ cups chopped spinach
- ½ cup ricotta cheese
- ½ tablespoon olives oil
- 2 small cloves garlic, peeled, minced

Directions:

1. Place an ovenproof, nonstick pan over medium heat. Add oil. When the oil is heated, add, onion and garlic and sauté until onion turns translucent.
2. Stir in the spinach and cook until it wilts.
3. Add rest of the ingredients into another bowl and whisk well. Pour into the skillet. Cook until the edges are set. Turn off the heat and transfer into an oven.
4. Bake in a preheated oven at 350° F for about 25 – 30 minutes

Omelet with Summer Vegetables

Number of servings: 2

Nutritional values per serving:

Calories – 187, Fat – 6 g, Carbohydrate – 11 g, Fiber – 1.6 g, Protein – 22 g, Sodium – 270 mg, Potassium – 352 mg, Phosphorous – 218 mg, Calcium – NA

Ingredients:

- ½ cup frozen corn kernels, thawed
- 6 tablespoons chopped green onions
- ½ teaspoon pepper or ½ teaspoon Extra spicy Mrs. Dash
- 2/3 cup chopped zucchini
- ¼ cup water
- 2 whole eggs
- 4 large egg whites
- 2 ounces shredded low-fat sharp cheddar cheese

Directions:

1.   Place a saucepan over medium-high flame. Spray with cooking spray.
2.   Add zucchini, corn and green onions and cook until the vegetables are crisp as well as tender. Turn off the heat.
3.   Whisk together in a bowl, eggs, whites, water, and seasoning.
4.   Place a small nonstick skillet over medium-high heat. Spray with cooking spray and let the pan heat.

5.   Pour half the egg mixture into the pan. When the edges begin to set, lift the edges of the omelet to let uncooked egg to go into the bottom of the pan.

6.   When the eggs are cooked, place half the vegetable mixture on one half of the omelet. Scatter half the cheese over the vegetables. Fold the other half of the omelet over the filling and cook for a couple of minutes.

7.   Remove onto a plate and serve.

8. Repeat steps 4-7 and make the other omelet.

Quick and Easy Apple Oatmeal Custard

Number of servings: 2

Nutritional values per serving:

Calories – 248, Fat – 8 g, Carbohydrate – 33 g, Fiber – 5.8 g, Protein – 11 g, Sodium – 164 mg, Potassium – 362 mg, Phosphorous – 240 mg, Calcium – 154 mg

Ingredients:

- 2/3 cup quick-cooking oatmeal
- 1 cup almond milk
- 1 medium apple, cored, finely chopped
- 2 large eggs
- ½ teaspoon ground cinnamon

Directions:

1. Add eggs and almond milk into a bowl and whisk well.
2. Add rest of the ingredients and stir well.
3. Place in the microwave and cook on high for 3 minutes. Stir once after 2 minutes of cooking.

Chapter 4: Lunch Recipes

Chicken Noodle Soup

Number of servings: 2

Nutritional values per serving:

Calories – 141, Fat – 4 g, Carbohydrate – 11 g, Fiber – 0.7 g, Protein – 15 g, Sodium – 191 mg, Potassium – 135 mg, Phosphorous – 104 mg, Calcium – 16 mg

Ingredients:

- ¾ cup low sodium chicken broth
- 1/8 teaspoon poultry seasoning
- A pinch salt
- Pepper to taste
- ½ cup cooked, shredded chicken
- 1 ounce egg noodles, uncooked
- ½ cup water
- 2 tablespoons chopped carrot

Directions:

1. Add all the ingredients into a soup pot. Place the pot over medium heat.
2. Cook until noodles are al dente.
3. Divide into 2 soup bowls and serve.

Cool Cucumber Soup

Number of servings: 10

Nutritional values per serving: ¾ cup

Calories – 77, Fat – 5 g, Carbohydrate – 6 g, Fiber – 1 g, Protein – 2 g, Sodium – 128 mg, Potassium – 258 mg, Phosphorous – 64 mg, Calcium – 60 mg

Ingredients:

- 4 medium cucumbers, peeled, deseeded, chopped
- 2 green onions, chopped
- ¼ cup fresh dill + extra to garnish
- ½ cup fresh mint leaves
- 2/3 cup sweet white onion, chopped
- 1 1/3 cups water
- ¼ cup lemon juice
- 1 cup half and half
- 1 teaspoon pepper
- 2/3 cup sour cream
- ½ teaspoon salt

Directions:

1. Gather all the ingredients and add into a blender.
2. Blend for 30 – 40 seconds or until smooth. Pour into a large bowl.
3. Cover and chill until use.
4. Ladle into soup bowls. Garnish with dill and serve.

BBQ Chicken Pita Pizza

Number of servings: 1

Nutritional values per serving:

Calories – 320, Fat – 9 g, Carbohydrate – 37 g, Fiber – 2.4 g, Protein – 23 g, Sodium – 523 mg, Potassium – 255 mg, Phosphorous – 221 mg, Calcium – 163 mg

Ingredients:

- 1 pita bread (6 ½ inches)
- 2 tablespoons chopped purple onion
- 2 ounces chicken, cooked
- 1 ½ tablespoons low-sodium BBQ☐sauce
- 1 tablespoon crumbled feta cheese
- A pinch garlic powder

Directions:

1. Grease a baking sheet with cooking spray.
2. Drizzle BBQ sauce over the pita and spread it evenly.
3. Scatter onion, chicken, garlic powder and feta cheese over the pitas.
4. Bake in a preheated oven at 350° F for about 25 – 30 minutes.
5. Serve hot.

Crunchy Quinoa Salad

Number of servings: 4

Nutritional values per serving:

Calories – 158, Fat – 9 g, Carbohydrate – 16 g, Fiber – 2.3 g, Protein – 5 g, Sodium – 46 mg, Potassium – 129 mg, Phosphorous – 237 mg, Calcium – 61 mg

Ingredients:

- ½ cup quinoa, rinsed, drained
- 2 ½ cherry tomatoes, diced
- 2 small green onions, chopped
- ¼ cup chopped, flat-leaf parsley
- ¼ cup diced cucumber (deseeded)
- 2 tablespoons chopped fresh mint
- 1 tablespoon fresh lemon juice
- 2 tablespoons olive oil
- 4 Bibb lettuce leaves, separated into cups
- ½ tablespoon grated lemon zest
- 2 tablespoons grated parmesan cheese

Directions:

1. Lightly toast the quinoa in a pan for about 2 to 3 minutes, over medium-high heat.
2. Pour water and stir. When it begins to boil, lower the heat and cover with a lid. Cook until dry. Using a fork, fluff the quinoa and let it cool.
3. Add rest of the ingredients except lettuce and Parmesan into a bowl and toss well. Add quinoa and toss well.

4. Divide into the lettuce cups. Garnish with Parmesan and serve.

Cool and Crispy Cucumber Salad

Number of servings: 2

Nutritional values per serving:

Calories – 27, Fat – 2 g, Carbohydrate – 3 g, Fiber – NA, Protein – NA, Sodium – 74 mg, Potassium – 90 mg, Phosphorous – 14 mg, Calcium – 12 mg

Ingredients:

- 1 cup chopped fresh cucumber (cut into ¼ inch thick slices, peel if desired)
- Freshly ground pepper to taste
- 1 tablespoon Italian or Caesar salad dressing

Directions:

1. Add cucumber and dressing into a bowl and toss well.
2. Garnish with pepper. Cover and chill until use.

Three-Pea Salad with Ginger-Lime Vinaigrette

Number of servings: 3

Nutritional values per serving:

Calories – 225, Fat – 21 g, Carbohydrate – 6 g, Fiber – 1.8 g, Protein – 3 g, Sodium – 70 mg, Potassium – 170 mg, Phosphorous – 40 mg, Calcium – 46 mg

Ingredients:

- ½ cup sugar snap peas
- ½ cup fresh or thawed frozen sweet peas
- ½ cup snow peas
- Freshly cracked pepper to garnish (optional)

For vinaigrette:

- ½ teaspoon low sodium soy sauce
- ½ teaspoon fresh lime zest
- ¼ cup canola oil
- ½ tablespoon sesame seeds, toasted
- 2 tablespoons fresh lime juice
- 1 teaspoon chopped, fresh ginger
- ½ tablespoon hot sesame oil

Directions:

1. Place a pot half-filled with water over high heat. When it begins to boil, add all the varieties of peas and cook for 2 minutes.
2. Drain and place the peas in a bowl of chilled water. Drain after 2-3 minutes and place in a bowl
3. Add all the ingredients for vinaigrette into a bowl and whisk well.

4. Pour dressing over the peas. Toss well. Garnish with pepper and serve.

Chicken Broccoli Stromboli

Number of servings: 2

Nutritional values per serving:

Calories – 522, Fat – 17 g, Carbohydrate – 52 g, Fiber – 2.9 g, Protein – 38 g, Sodium – 607 mg, Potassium – 546 mg, Phosphorous – 400 mg, Calcium – 262 mg

Ingredients:

- ½ pound store-bought pizza dough
- 1 cup cooked, diced chicken breast
- ½ tablespoon chopped garlic
- ½ teaspoon crushed red pepper flakes
- 1 tablespoon olive oil
- 1 cup broccoli florets, blanched
- ½ cup shredded, low salt mozzarella cheese
- ½ tablespoon chopped, fresh oregano
- 1 tablespoon flour

Directions:

1. Add chicken, red pepper flakes, garlic, cheese, broccoli, and oregano into a bowl and toss well.
2. Sprinkle 1-tablespoon flour on your countertop. Place the dough on your countertop and roll into a rectangle with a rolling pin (about 5 x 7 inches).
3. Place the filling on the longer part of the dough, leaving 2 inches border. Roll the dough and seal the ends by pressing and finally crimp the edges with a fork.

4. Brush oil on top. Make 2-3 small slits on the dough (on top) for the steam to escape.
5. Bake in a preheated oven at 400° F for about 25 – 30 minutes.

Egg Fried Rice

Number of servings: 5

Nutritional values per serving: 1 cup

Calories – 137, Fat – 4 g, Carbohydrate – 21 g, Fiber – 1.3 g, Protein – 5 g, Sodium – 38 mg, Potassium – 89 mg, Phosphorous – 67 mg, Calcium – 20 mg

Ingredients:

- 1 teaspoon dark sesame oil
- 1 egg white
- 1 whole egg
- ½ tablespoon canola oil
- 1 green onion, chopped (about 3 tablespoons)
- ½ cup frozen peas, thawed
- ½ cup bean sprouts
- 2 cups, cooked, cold rice
- 1/8 teaspoon pepper

Directions:

1. Add sesame oil, egg white and whole egg into a bowl and whisk well.
2. Place a nonstick pan over medium-high heat. Add canola oil. When the oil is heated, add egg mixture and frequently stir until the eggs are cooked.
3. Stir in the green onion and bean sprouts. Cook for 2 minutes.
4. Add rice, peas and pepper and heat thoroughly.
5. Serve right away.

Hawaiian Chicken Salad Sandwich

Number of servings: 2

Nutritional values per serving: 1-cup chicken salad with 1 tortilla

Calories – 349, Fat – 17 g, Carbohydrate – 24 g, Fiber – 1.5 g, Protein – 22 g, Sodium – 398 mg, Potassium – 333 mg, Phosphorous – 167 mg, Calcium – 15 mg

Ingredients:

- 1 cup cooked, shredded chicken
- ¼ cup low-fat mayonnaise
- 3 tablespoons chopped carrots
- 2 pieces flatbread or flour tortillas (6 inches each)
- ½ cup pineapple tidbits, drained
- ¼ cup chopped green bell pepper
- ¼ teaspoon pepper

Directions:

1. Add all the ingredients except flatbreads into a bowl and toss well.
2. Chill until use.
3. Divide the salad among the flatbread or tortillas (place over flatbread if using or roll if using tortilla and serve).

Tortilla Beef Rollups

Number of servings: 1

Nutritional values per serving:

Calories – 258, Fat – 10 g, Carbohydrate – 18 g, Fiber – 1.6 g, Protein – 24 g, Sodium – 279 mg, Potassium – 448 mg, Phosphorous – 253 mg, Calcium – 59 mg

Ingredients:

- 1 flour tortilla (6 inches)
- 2.5 ounces roast beef, cooked
- 1/8 bell pepper or any color, cut into strips
- 1 romaine lettuce leaves
- 1 tablespoon whipped cream cheese
- 2 tablespoons chopped red onion
- 4 cucumber slices
- ½ teaspoon Mrs. Dash herb seasoning blend

Directions:

1. Place the tortilla on a plate and spread cream cheese all over it.
2. Scatter beef all over the tortilla followed by the vegetables. Season with Mrs. Dash herb seasoning.
3. Roll the tortilla along with the filling and place with its seam side facing down on a plate and serve.

Macaroni and Cheese

Number of servings: 2

Nutritional values per serving:

Calories – 163, Fat – 7 g, Carbohydrate – 20 g, Fiber – 3 g, Protein – 6 g, Sodium – 114 mg, Potassium – 39 mg, Phosphorous – 138 mg, Calcium – 120 mg

Ingredients:

- 1 cup elbow pasta
- ¼ cup grated cheddar cheese
- 1/8 teaspoon dried mustard
- 1 ½ -2 cups water
- ½ teaspoon margarine or unsalted butter

Directions:

1. Add water into a pot and place over high heat. Add pasta and cook until al dente. Drain and place in a bowl.
2. Add rest of the ingredients and toss well.
3. Serve hot.

Shrimp Quesadilla

Number of servings: 1

Nutritional values per serving:

Calories – 318, Fat – 15 g, Carbohydrate – 26 g, Fiber – 1.2 g, Protein – 20 g, Sodium – 398 mg, Potassium – 276 mg, Phosphorous – 243 mg, Calcium – 139 mg

Ingredients:

- 2.5 ounces raw shrimp, shelled, deveined, cut into bite-size pieces
- ½ tablespoon lemon juice
- A pinch cayenne pepper
- 1 tablespoon sour cream
- 1 tablespoon shredded, jalapeño cheddar cheese
- 1 tablespoon chopped cilantro
- 1/8 teaspoon ground cumin
- 1 flour tortilla (10 inches)
- 2 teaspoons salsa

Directions:

1. Add cilantro, cumin, lemon juice, and cayenne pepper into a Ziploc bag. Shake the bag until well combined. Add shrimp and seal the bag. Turn the bag around a few times until shrimp is well coated. Let it sit for 5 minutes.
2. Place a skillet over medium heat. Add shrimp along with the marinade and sauté until shrimp becomes orange in color. Turn off the heat.
3. Remove shrimp with a slotted spoon and set aside.

4. Add sour cream into the skillet with remaining marinade and mix well.
5. Heat the tortilla following the direction on the package.
6. Place the tortilla on a plate. Spread salsa over the tortilla. Place shrimp on one half of the tortilla. Top shrimp with cheese.
7. Spread 1 tablespoon of the marinade mixture over the shrimp. Fold the other half of the tortilla over the filling. Press slightly.
8. Cook until the underside is golden brown. Flip sides and cook the other side until golden brown.

Chapter 5: Dinner Recipes
Herb-Roasted Chicken Breasts

Number of servings: 2

Nutritional values per serving:

Calories – 270, Fat – 17 g, Carbohydrate – 3 g, Fiber – 0.6 g, Protein – 26 g, Sodium – 53 mg, Potassium – 491 mg, Phosphorous – 252 mg, Calcium – 17 mg

Ingredients:

- ½ pound skinless, boneless chicken breasts
- 1 clove garlic, minced
- ½ teaspoon pepper
- 1 small onion, chopped
- 1 tablespoon Mrs. Dash Garlic and Herb seasoning blend
- 2 tablespoons olive oil

Directions:

1. Add all the ingredients except chicken into a bowl and mix until well combined.
2. Add chicken and turn it around in the marinade a few times until well coated.
3. Cover and chill for 4 – 8 hours.
4. Line a baking sheet with foil and place the chicken pieces on it. Drizzle the marinade over the chicken.
5. Bake in a preheated oven at 400° F for about 20 minutes.
6. Set the oven to broil mode and broil the chicken until brown on both sides.

Chicken Pot Pie Stew

Number of servings: 4

Nutritional values per serving:

Calories – 388, Fat – 21 g, Carbohydrate – 22 g, Fiber – 2 g, Protein – 26 g, Sodium – 424 mg, Potassium – 209 mg, Phosphorous – 290 mg, Calcium – 88 mg

Ingredients:

- ¾ pound skinless, boneless, fresh chicken breast, pound with a meat mallet, cut into pieces
- 2 tablespoons canola oil
- ¼ cup chopped carrots
- 2 tablespoons chopped celery
- ¼ cup chopped onion
- ¼ teaspoon pepper
- 1 teaspoon Better than bouillon, low sodium chicken base
- ¼ cup heavy cream
- ½ cup low-fat, grated cheddar cheese
- 1 cup low-sodium chicken stock
- ¼ cup flour
- ½ tablespoon sodium-free Italian seasoning like McCormick
- ¼ cup frozen sweet peas, thawed
- ½ frozen pie crust, baked, broken into bite-size pieces

Directions:

1. Add chicken and stock into a pot and place over medium-high heat. Let it cook for about 20 minutes.
2. Add oil and flour into a bowl and mix well. Add into the simmering pot of chicken.
3. Stir constantly until slightly thick. Lower the heat and continue simmering for 8-10 minutes.
4. Stir in carrot, celery, onion, bouillon, and seasonings. Simmer for another 10 minutes. Remove from heat.
5. Add peas and cream and mix well.
6. Divide into 4 mugs. Divide the cheese and piecrusts among the mugs and serve.

Honey Garlic Chicken

Number of servings: 2

Nutritional values per serving:

Calories – 279, Fat – 10 g, Carbohydrate – 36 g, Fiber – 0 g, Protein – 13 g, Sodium – 40 mg, Potassium – 144 mg, Phosphorous – 99 mg, Calcium – 11 mg

Ingredients:

- 2 pounds roasting chicken, cut into pieces
- ½ teaspoon garlic powder
- ½ tablespoon olive oil, to grease
- ¼ cup honey
- ¼ teaspoon pepper

Directions:

1. Grease a baking dish with olive oil. Place chicken in the baking dish, in a single layer.
2. Brush with honey all over the chicken. Sprinkle garlic powder and pepper.
3. Bake in a preheated oven at 350° F for about 45 minutes or until brown and cooked through. Flip sides halfway through baking.
4. Serve hot.

Chicken Veronique

Number of servings: 1

Nutritional values per serving:

Calories – 306, Fat – 18 g, Carbohydrate – 9 g, Fiber – 0.5 g, Protein – 27 g, Sodium –167 mg, Potassium – 543 mg, Phosphorous – 292 mg, Calcium – 52 mg

Ingredients:

- 1 chicken breast, skinless, boneless (4 ounces)
- 1 tablespoon butter
- 1 tablespoon low-sodium chicken broth
- ½ teaspoon dried tarragon
- ¼ shallot, finely chopped
- 1 tablespoon dry white wine
- ¼ cup seedless green grapes
- 2 tablespoons cream

Directions:

1. Place a skillet over medium heat. Add butter. When butter melts, add chicken and cook until golden brown all over. Remove with a slotted spoon and place on a plate lined with paper towels.
2. Add shallot into the skillet and cook until soft.
3. Add cornstarch, broth, and wine into a bowl and whisk well. Add into the skillet and constantly stir until thick.
4. Add chicken and coat it well with the sauce.

5. Lower the heat and cover with a lid. Simmer until chicken is cooked through. Remove onto a serving plate.
6. Add cream and tarragon into the same skillet.
7. When it begins to boil, add grapes and heat thoroughly.
8. Pour over the chicken and serve.

Barley and Beef Stew

Number of servings: 3

Nutritional values per serving: 1-¼ cups

Calories – 246, Fat – 8 g, Carbohydrate – 21 g, Fiber – 6.3 g, Protein – 22 g, Sodium – 222 mg, Potassium – 369 mg, Phosphorous – 175 mg, Calcium – 30 mg

Ingredients:

- ½ cup pearl barley, rinsed, soaked in a cup for water for an hour, drained
- 1 tablespoon all-purpose white flour
- ¼ teaspoon salt
- ¼ cup chopped onion
- 2 small cloves garlic, peeled, sliced
- 1 medium carrot, cut into ¼ inch thick pieces
- ½ teaspoon Mrs. Dash onion herb seasoning
- ½ pound lean beef stew meat, cut into ½ inch pieces
- 1/8 teaspoon pepper
- 1 tablespoon canola oil
- 1 medium stalk celery, chopped
- ½ teaspoon Mrs. Dash onion herb seasoning
- 1 bay leaf
- 4 cups water or more if required

Directions:

1. Add flour and pepper into a bowl and stir.
2. Place meat in a bowl and sprinkle the flour mixture over it and toss until well coated.

3. Place a soup pot over medium heat. Add oil. When the oil is heated, add meat and cook until brown. Remove with a slotted spoon and place on a plate.
4. Add onion, garlic, and celery into the pot and cook until onion turns translucent.
5. Add water and stir.
6. When it begins to boil, add meat, salt and bay leaves and stir.
7. Lower the heat. Add barley and stir. Cover with a lid and simmer for about 45 minutes. Stir occasionally.
8. Add carrot and seasoning and cook for 40-45 minutes or until barley and carrots are cooked. Add more water if required.
9. Ladle into bowls and serve.

Chili Con Carne

Number of servings: 4

Nutritional values per serving: 1 cup

Calories – 190, Fat – 10 g, Carbohydrate – 5 g, Fiber – 1.25 g, Protein – 20 g, Sodium – 116 mg, Potassium – 450 mg, Phosphorous – 180 mg, Calcium – 38 mg

Ingredients:

- ¼ cup chopped onion
- ¼ cup chopped green bell pepper
- 8 ounces low-sodium stewed tomatoes, blended
- 1 tablespoon chili powder
- ½ stalk celery, chopped
- ¾ pound lean ground beef
- ½ tablespoon canola oil
- ¾ cup water

Directions:

1. Place a skillet over medium heat. Add oil. When the oil is heated, add onion, bell pepper, and celery and cook until slightly soft.
2. Stir in the beef and cook until brown. Break it simultaneously as it cooks.
3. Add tomatoes, chili powder, and water and stir.
4. Lower the heat. Cover and cook for 1 – 1-½ hours and stir occasionally.

Curried Turkey and Rice

Number of servings: 3

Nutritional values per serving:

Calories – 154, Fat – 5 g, Carbohydrate – 20 g, Fiber – 1 g, Protein – 8 g, Sodium – 27 mg, Potassium – 156 mg, Phosphorous – 88 mg, Calcium – 25 mg

Ingredients:

- ½ teaspoon vegetable oil
- 1 small onion, chopped
- 1 teaspoon curry powder
- ½ cup low-sodium chicken broth
- ½ teaspoon sugar
- ½ pound turkey breast, cut into 3 cutlets
- ½ tablespoon unsalted margarine
- 1 tablespoon flour
- ¼ cup non-dairy creamer
- 1 cup cooked white rice

Directions:

1. Place a skillet over medium heat. Add turkey and cook until it is not pink anymore.
2. Remove onto a plate. Cover turkey with aluminum foil.
3. Add margarine into the skillet. When it melts, add onion and stir for a couple of minutes. Add curry powder and sauté for 2-3 minutes.

4. Stir in the flour. Stir constantly for a minute. Add broth, sugar, and creamer, stirring constantly. Keep stirring until thick.
5. Add turkey and mix well. Heat thoroughly.
6. Divide rice into 3 plates. Place 1 cutlet on each plate, over the rice. Divide the gravy and spoon over the cutlets.
7. Serve immediately.

Spicy Pork Chops with Apples

Number of servings: 3

Nutritional values per serving: Without rice

Calories – 215, Fat – 13 g, Carbohydrate – 9.8 g, Fiber – NA, Protein – 15 g, Sodium – 330 mg, Potassium – 288 mg, Phosphorous – 126 mg, Calcium – NA

Ingredients:

- 1 clove garlic, peeled, minced
- ½ teaspoon ground ginger
- 1/8 teaspoon pepper
- ¼ teaspoon + 1/8 teaspoon salt
- ¼ teaspoon sugar
- 1/8 teaspoon ground cumin
- 1 medium apple, cored, cut into 1 inch thick slices
- 3 large pork chops
- 1 medium onion, cut into ¾ inch thick wedges

Directions:

1. Add all the spices, sugar, and salt into a bowl and stir.
2. Rub this mixture all over the pork chops and place in a small, glass baking dish.
3. Place apple slices and onion slices in between the pork pieces.
4. Crumple some foil and place all around the inner sides of the dish so that the pork, onion and apple and sticking together.
5. Cover the dish with another sheet of foil.

6. Bake in a preheated oven at 400° F for about 30 – 35 minutes.
7. Remove the foil on the top as well as the ones inside the dish and separate the apples, onion and pork chops.
8. Bake for another 15 minutes or until light brown on top.
9. Divide into 3 equal portions and serve over rice.

Irish Lamb Stew

Number of servings: 3

Nutritional values per serving:

Calories – 283, Fat – 11 g, Carbohydrate – 19 g, Fiber – 3.4 g, Protein – 27 g, Sodium – 325 mg, Potassium – 527 mg, Phosphorous – 300 mg, Calcium – 56 mg

Ingredients:

- ¾ pound boneless lamb shoulder, chopped into bite-size chunks
- ¼ teaspoon pepper
- ¼ teaspoon salt
- ½ tablespoon olive oil
- 2 tablespoons all-purpose flour
- ½ teaspoon dried thyme
- ½ cup stout beer
- 1 medium carrot, cubed (1 inch)
- ½ cup frozen peas
- 1 medium parsnip, cubed (1 inch)
- 1 small onion, chopped
- 2 cloves garlic, minced
- ¼ cup tomato sauce
- 1 cup low-sodium beef broth

Directions:

1. Season lamb with salt and pepper. Sprinkle flour all over the lamb and toss well.

2. Place a soup pot over medium heat. Add oil. When the oil is heated, add lamb and cook until brown all over. Remove with a slotted spoon and set aside.
3. Add onions into the pot and cook until pink. Add garlic and stir-fry for a few seconds until aromatic.
4. Add broth and scrape the bottom of the pot to remove any browned bits that may be stuck.
5. Stir in lamb, beer, thyme, and tomato sauce. When it begins to boil, lower the heat and simmer for about 30 to 40 minutes.
6. Add carrots and parsnips and mix well. Cover and cook until tender.
7. Add peas and simmer for another 10 minutes.
8. Ladle into bowls and serve.

Marinated Shrimp

Number of servings: 6

Nutritional values per serving: 6 shrimp

Calories – 188, Fat – 12 g, Carbohydrate – 2.4 g, Fiber – NA, Protein – 17 g, Sodium – 180 mg, Potassium – 187 mg, Phosphorous – 162 mg, Calcium – NA

Ingredients:

- 1 ¼ pounds large shrimp
- 6 tablespoons vinegar
- ½ teaspoon salt
- ¾ teaspoon celery seeds
- 2 small cloves garlic, peeled, minced
- 1 cup thinly sliced onions
- ¾ cup oil
- 1 heaping teaspoon capers with a little liquid
- ½ teaspoon whole cloves
- A dash red pepper sauce
- 4 bay leaves

Directions:

1. Place shrimp in a baking dish. Scatter onions over it. Place bay leaves on top.
2. Add rest of the ingredients into a bowl and whisk well. Pour over the shrimp and onions.
3. Chill for at least 24 hours.
4. Serve chilled.

Shrimp & Coconut Curry Noodle Bowl

Number of servings: 10

Nutritional values per serving:

Calories – 418, Fat – 27 g, Carbohydrate – 36 g, Fiber – 5 g, Protein – 16 g, Sodium – 195 mg, Potassium – 660 mg, Phosphorous – 285 mg, Calcium – 90 mg

Ingredients:

- 16 ounces rice noodles
- 2 sweet onions, diced
- 4 ears sweet corn, use kernels
- 2 tablespoons freshly grated ginger
- 4 cloves garlic, peeled, minced
- 6 tablespoons Thai red curry paste or to taste
- 2/3 – 1 cup water
- 4 teaspoons honey
- 2 tablespoons low-sodium soy sauce
- Juice of a lime
- Zest of a lime, grated
- 4 tablespoons coconut oil
- 4 zucchini, diced
- 2 cans (14 ounces each) full fat coconut milk

For topping:

- A handful fresh cilantro, chopped
- 1 jalapeño pepper, sliced
- 1 green onion, thinly sliced

Directions:

1. Follow the instructions on the package and cook the noodles. Set aside.
2. Place a large skillet over high heat. Add oil. When the oil is heated, add onions and stir-fry for 4-5 minutes.
3. Stir in the corn, zucchini, garlic, and ginger and cook until slightly tender.
4. Add curry paste and stir-fry for 50-60 seconds.
5. Add rest of the ingredients except lime juice and zest and mix well. Add more water if required. Heat thoroughly. Turn off the heat.
6. Add lime juice and zest and stir.
7. Divide the noodles into 10 bowls. Divide the curry and spoon over the noodles.
8. Top with suggested toppings and serve.

Seafood Corn Chowder

Number of servings: 5

Nutritional values per serving:

Calories – 173, Fat – 7 g, Carbohydrate – 22 g, Fiber – 1.5 g, Protein – 8 g, Sodium – 160 mg, Potassium – 258 mg, Phosphorous – 181 mg, Calcium – 68 mg

Ingredients:

- ½ tablespoon unsalted butter
- 3 tablespoons chopped celery
- ¼ cup chopped red bell pepper
- ¼ cup chopped green bell pepper
- ½ cup chopped onion
- ½ tablespoon all-purpose white flour
- 1 cup liquid nondairy creamer
- 5 ounces surimi imitation crab chunks
- ¼ teaspoon pepper
- 7 ounces low-sodium chicken broth
- 3 ounces evaporated milk
- 1 cup frozen corn kernels
- ¼ teaspoon paprika

Directions:

1. Place a soup pot over medium heat. Add butter. When butter melts, add onion, bell peppers and celery and cook until tender.
2. Stir in the flour. Keep stirring for a couple of minutes.

3. Add broth, stirring constantly. Keep stirring until slightly thick.
4. Add rest of the ingredients and stir. Heat thoroughly.
5. Ladle into bowls and serve.

Spaghetti and Asparagus Carbonara

Number of servings: 3

Nutritional values per serving: 1 cup

Calories – 304, Fat – 19 g, Carbohydrate – 27 g, Fiber – 5.4 g, Protein – 9 g, Sodium – 9 mg, Potassium – 287 mg, Phosphorous – 143 mg, Calcium – 95 mg

Ingredients:

- 1 teaspoon canola oil
- 1 small egg, beaten
- 2 tablespoons low-sodium chicken stock
- 1 cup fresh, chopped asparagus (1 inch pieces)
- ¼ cup chopped scallions
- 1 ½ tablespoons shredded parmesan cheese
- ½ cup diced onions
- ½ cup heavy cream
- 1 ½ cups cooked spiral noodle pasta
- ½ teaspoon freshly cracked coarse pepper
- 1 ½ tablespoons meatless bacon bits

Directions:

1. Place a nonstick pan over medium-high heat. Add oil. When the oil is heated, add onion and cook until light brown. Reduce the heat to medium heat.
2. Add egg and cream into a bowl and whisk well. Pour into the pan and keep stirring until egg begins to set.
3. Stir in asparagus, stock, pepper, and pasta. Heat thoroughly, stirring constantly. Remove from heat.

4. Divide into 3 plates. Divide the scallions, cheese and bacon bits equally and sprinkle over the pasta.
5. Serve hot.

Chapter 6: Side Dishes

Italian Eggplant Salad

Number of servings: 2

Nutritional values per serving: ½ cup

Calories – 69, Fat – 5 g, Carbohydrate – 6 g, Fiber – NA, Protein – 1 g, Sodium – 2 mg, Potassium – 118 mg, Phosphorous – 15 mg, Calcium – 10 mg

Ingredients:

- 1 ½ cups cubed eggplant
- 1 tablespoon white wine vinegar
- ¼ teaspoon oregano
- 1 small tomato, chopped
- ½ small onion, chopped
- 2 small cloves garlic, chopped
- 1/8 teaspoon pepper
- 1 ½ tablespoons olive oil

Directions:

1. Half fill a small saucepan with water and place over high heat. When it begins to boil, add eggplant. When it begins to boil again, lower the heat and cook until tender.
2. Drain off the water from the eggplant and place in a glass dish.
3. Add onion and stir.

4. Add vinegar, pepper, and garlic into a bowl and whisk well. Drizzle over the eggplant mixture. Stir well.
5. Add oil just before serving. Stir and serve.

Sautéed Collard Greens

Number of servings: 3

Nutritional values per serving:

Calories – 79, Fat – 7 g, Carbohydrate – 4 g, Fiber – 2.2 g, Protein – 2 g, Sodium – 9 mg, Potassium – 129 mg, Phosphorous – 18 mg, Calcium – 118 mg

Ingredients:

- 4 cups chopped, fresh collard greens
- ½ tablespoon unsalted butter
- ½ tablespoon chopped garlic
- ½ teaspoon pepper
- 1 tablespoon olive oil
- 2 tablespoons finely chopped onions
- ½ teaspoon crushed red pepper flakes
- ½ tablespoon vinegar (optional)

Directions:

1. Place a saucepan half-filled with water over high heat. When it begins to boil, add collard greens and drain off after exactly 30 seconds.
2. Drain and place in a bowl of chilled water. Drain off after 5-6 minutes.
3. Place a skillet over medium-high heat. Add butter and oil. When the butter melts, add garlic and onions and sauté until light brown.
4. Raise the heat to high heat. Stir in the collard greens, red pepper flakes, and pepper and cook for 4-5 minutes. Turn off the heat.

5. Add vinegar if using and toss well.
6. Serve hot.

BBQ Asparagus

Number of servings: 3

Nutritional values per serving:

Calories – 86, Fat – 6 g, Carbohydrate – 5 g, Fiber – 2 g, Protein – 3 g, Sodium – 4 mg, Potassium – 196 mg, Phosphorous – 41 mg, Calcium – 20 mg

Ingredients:

- ¾ pound fresh asparagus, trimmed
- ¾ teaspoon pepper
- 1 ½ tablespoons extra-virgin olive oil
- 1 ½ tablespoons lemon juice

Directions:

1. Add oil, lemon juice, and pepper into a shallow, wide dish. Place the asparagus in the bowl. Turn it around so that the asparagus is well coated with the mixture.
2. Chill until you prepare the grill.
3. Preheat a gas grill or charcoal grill to medium-high heat. Spray some cooking spray inside the grill basket or line (aluminum foil) and grease a vegetable-grilling tray.
4. Place the asparagus in the grill tray or basket and grill until light brown. Stir frequently.
5. Remove onto a plate. Cool for a couple of minutes and serve.

Crunchy Green Bean Casserole

Number of servings: 3

Nutritional values per serving:

Calories – 122, Fat – 6 g, Carbohydrate – 11 g, Fiber – 2.4 g, Protein – 4 g, Sodium – 221 mg, Potassium – 219 mg, Phosphorous – 49 mg, Calcium – 88 mg

Ingredients:

- 6 ounces fresh string green beans, cut into 2 inch pieces
- 2 tablespoons crumbled gorgonzola or sharp cheddar cheese
- ¼ cup panko breadcrumbs
- ¼ cup plain unsalted tortilla chips, crushed
- 1 tablespoon hot sauce
- 1 tablespoon unsalted butter, melted
- 1 tablespoon chopped green onions

Directions:

1. Place beans in a microwave-safe bowl and cook on high for about 4 -5 minutes.
2. Add hot sauce and toss well.
3. Transfer into a small casserole dish.
4. Add rest of the ingredients into a bowl and stir. Sprinkle over the beans.
5. Bake in a preheated oven at 375° F for about 12 – 15 minutes.

Mediterranean Green Beans

Number of servings: 2

Nutritional values per serving: 1 cup

Calories – 71, Fat – 3 g, Carbohydrate – 10 g, Fiber – 3.7 g, Protein – 2 g, Sodium – 2 mg, Potassium – 186 mg, Phosphorous – 37 mg, Calcium – 55 mg

Ingredients:

- ½ pound fresh green beans, trimmed, cut into 1 ½ inch pieces
- 1 ¼ teaspoons olive oil
- 1 ½ tablespoons fresh lemon juice
- 6 tablespoons water
- 2 cloves garlic, peeled, minced
- A pinch pepper

Directions:

1. Add water into a skillet. Place over medium-high heat. When it begins to boil, add beans and let it boil for 3 minutes. Drain in a colander.
2. Place the skillet back over heat. Add oil. When the oil is heated, add beans and garlic and cook for a minute.
3. Stir in the juice and pepper stir-fry for a minute.
4. Serve hot.

Chapter 7: Snack Recipes

Cranberry Dip with Fresh Fruit

Number of servings: 6

Nutritional values per serving: 2 tablespoons dip with 3 pineapple chunks and 2 slices each of pear and apple

Calories – 70, Fat – 2 g, Carbohydrate – 13 g, Fiber – 1.5 g, Protein – 0 g, Sodium – 8 mg, Potassium – 101 mg, Phosphorous – 15 mg, Calcium – 17 mg

Ingredients:

- 2 ounces sour cream
- A pinch ground nutmeg
- 1 cup chopped pineapple chunks
- 1 medium pear, cored, peeled, cut into 12 slices
- ¼ teaspoon lemon juice
- 2 tablespoons whole berry cranberry sauce
- A pinch ground ginger
- 1 medium apple, cored, cut into 12 slices

Directions:

1. Add apple and pear into a bowl. Drizzle lemon juice over it and toss well.
2. Place apple, pear and pineapple slices on a serving platter.
3. Add rest of the ingredients into the small blender jar. Blend until smooth.
4. Pour into a bowl. Chill the dip and fruits until use.

Cucumbers with Sour Cream

Number of servings: 2

Nutritional values per serving: ½ cup

Calories – 64, Fat – 5 g, Carbohydrate – 4 g, Fiber – 0.8 g, Protein – 1 g, Sodium – 72 mg, Potassium – 113 mg, Phosphorous – 24 mg, Calcium – 21 mg

Ingredients:

- 1 medium cucumber, peeled, thinly sliced
- ¼ medium sweet onion, thinly sliced
- A pinch salt (less than 1/8 teaspoon)
- 2 tablespoons white wine vinegar
- A pinch pepper
- ½ tablespoon canola oil
- ¼ cup low-fat sour cream

Directions:

1. Place cucumber slices in a bowl. Sprinkle salt and toss well. Squeeze the cucumber of excess moisture after 15 minutes. Place in a bowl.
2. Add rest of the ingredients and toss well.
3. Refrigerate until use.
4. Serve chilled.

Spicy Corn Bread

Number of servings: 16

Nutritional values per serving: 2x4 inches piece

Calories – 188, Fat – 5 g, Carbohydrate – 31 g, Fiber – 2 g, Protein – 5 g, Sodium – 155 mg, Potassium – 100 mg, Phosphorous – 81 mg, Calcium – 84 mg

Ingredients:

For dry ingredients:

- 2 cups all-purpose white flour
- 2 tablespoons sugar
- 2 teaspoons chili powder
- 2 cups plain cornmeal
- 4 teaspoons baking powder
- ½ teaspoon pepper

For wet ingredients:

- 2 cups rice milk, un-enriched
- 2 egg whites
- 2 whole eggs
- 4 tablespoons canola oil
- ½ cup finely grated carrots
- 1 cup finely chopped scallions
- 2 cloves garlic, peeled, minced

Directions:

1. Add all the dry ingredients into a large mixing bowl and mix until well incorporated.

2. Add all the wet ingredients except the vegetables into the bowl of dry ingredients and mix well.
3. Add vegetables and stir.
4. Grease a large baking dish (9x13 inches) with cooking spray. Spoon the batter into the dish.
5. Bake in a preheated oven at 400° F for about 30 minutes or until the top begins to look golden brown.
6. Remove from the oven and cool on a wire rack.
7. Cut into 16 equal pieces of (2 x 4 inches) and serve.

Wonton Quiche Minis

Number of servings: 24

Nutritional values per serving: 2 wontons

Calories – 70, Fat – 4 g, Carbohydrate – 8 g, Fiber – 0.2 g, Protein – 4 g, Sodium – 95 mg, Potassium – 47 mg, Phosphorous – 55 mg, Calcium – 16 mg

Ingredients:

- 2 ounces lean cooked ham, finely chopped
- ¼ cup chopped sweet red bell pepper
- 2 tablespoon all-purpose white flour
- ¼ cup chopped green onion
- 10 large eggs
- 48 wonton wrappers (3 ¼ x3 inches)

Directions:

1. Add eggs into a bowl and whisk well. Add rest of the ingredients except wonton wrappers and whisk well.
2. Grease 48 mini muffin cups with cooking spray. Line each of the muffin cups with a wonton wrapper. Press it well into the cups, on the bottom as well as the sides of the cup.
3. Divide the egg mixture equally among the muffin cups.
4. Bake in a preheated oven at 400° F for about 12- 15 minutes. If the muffins are ready, a toothpick when inserted in the middle of muffins should come out clean without any particles.

5. Let it cool for a few minutes in the pan. Remove along with the wrappers and serve.

Buffalo Chicken Dip

Number of servings: 8

Nutritional values per serving: ¼ cup without vegetables

Calories – 73, Fat – 5 g, Carbohydrate – 2 g, Fiber – 0 g, Protein – 5 g, Sodium – 66 mg, Potassium – 81 mg, Phosphorous – 47 mg, Calcium – 31 mg

Ingredients:

- 2 ounces cream cheese
- ½ cup reduced-fat sour cream
- 1 cup cooked, shredded chicken
- ¼ cup bottled roasted red peppers, drained
- 2 teaspoons Tabasco hot pepper sauce

Directions:

1. Add red pepper into the small blender jar and blend until smooth. Transfer into a baking dish.
2. Add cream cheese, sour cream and Tabasco sauce into the baking dish
3. Add chicken and mix until well coated.
4. Bake in a preheated oven at 350° F for about 30 minutes or until chicken is cooked through. You can also cook it on a low setting in a slow cooker.
5. Serve with vegetables sticks like carrot, cucumber, etc.

Cran-Apple Cinnamon Snack Mix

Number of servings: 6

Nutritional values per serving: ¾ cup

Calories – 214, Fat – 2 g, Carbohydrate – 46 g, Fiber – 3.1 g, Protein – 3 g, Sodium – 159 mg, Potassium – 118 mg, Phosphorous – 67 mg, Calcium – 84 mg

Ingredients:

- ½ cup dried apples, chopped
- 1 cup Rice Chex cereal
- 1 cup Corn Chex cereal
- 1 ½ cups cinnamon Chex cereal
- 1 cup shredded wheat bite-size cereal
- ½ cup dried, sweetened cranberries
- ¼ cup sugar
- ½ teaspoon ground cinnamon
- 2 tablespoons liquid egg whites
- 1 tablespoon apple juice
- ½ tablespoon sesame seeds

Directions:

1. Grease a baking dish with cooking spray.
2. Add all the cereals, apple and cranberries into a bowl and toss well.
3. Add whites, apple juice, sugar, and cinnamon into another bowl and whisk well with an electric hand mixer until frothy.
4. Pour over the cereal mixture and stir until well coated.

5. Scatter sesame seeds and toss well. Spread it all over the dish.
6. Bake in a preheated oven at 300° F for about 30 – 45 minutes or until light brown and crisp. Stir every 12 – 15 minutes.
7. Let it cool to room temperature. Transfer into an airtight container and store until use.

Corn and Cheese Balls

Number of servings: 4

Nutritional values per serving: 4 balls

Calories – 253, Fat – 13 g, Carbohydrate – 27 g, Fiber – 2.3 g, Protein – 7 g, Sodium – 287 mg, Potassium – 169 mg, Phosphorous – 86 mg, Calcium – 46 mg

Ingredients:

- 1 cup frozen yellow corn, thawed
- 1 tablespoon chopped cilantro
- 2 slices white bread
- ½ teaspoon chili powder
- ½ teaspoon ground coriander
- ½ teaspoon ground cumin
- 1/8 teaspoon salt
- ½ green chili, minced
- ¼ cup cottage cheese
- ¼ cup all-purpose white flour
- 1 ½ cups vegetable oil

Directions:

1. Add cheese, corn, flour, cilantro, salt, and all the spices into a bowl and mix well.
2. Add some water into a bowl. Dip the bread slices in it for 10 – 15 seconds. Squeeze out as much water as possible from the bread slices.
3. Add into the corn mixture. Mix well.
4. Divide the mixture into 16 equal portions and shape into balls.

5. Place a deep pan with oil over medium heat. When the oil is well heated but not smoking, carefully drop 4-5 cornballs in the pan. Cook until golden brown all over.
6. Remove with a slotted spoon and place on a plate lined with paper towels.
7. Fry the remaining balls in batches similarly.
8. Serve hot.

Fresh Berry Fruit Salad with Yogurt Cream

Number of servings: 4

Nutritional values per serving:

Calories – 117, Fat – 0.4 g, Carbohydrate – 27 g, Fiber – 3 g, Protein – 3.7 g, Sodium – 40 mg, Potassium – 252 mg, Phosphorous – 90 mg, Calcium – NA

Ingredients:

For berry salad:

- 1 tablespoon honey
- ½ cup red cherries, pitted, halved
- ½ cup raspberries
- ½ cup blackberries
- ½ cup blueberries

For yogurt cream:

- 1 cup Greek yogurt
- ½ tablespoon lemon juice
- 2 tablespoons honey

Directions:

1. For the salad: Add berries into a bowl. Drizzle honey over it and toss well.
2. To make yogurt cream: Add all the ingredients for yogurt cream into a bowl and whisk well.
3. Divide the yogurt cream among 4 plates. Spread it in the center of the plate. Divide the berries and place over the yogurt.
4. Serve.

Chapter 8: Dessert Recipes

Apple and Blueberry Crisp

Number of servings: 4

Nutritional values per serving:

Calories – 318, Fat – 12 g, Carbohydrate – 52 g, Fiber – 4 g, Protein – 3.3 g, Sodium – 148 mg, Potassium – 196 mg, Phosphorous – 93 mg, Calcium – NA

Ingredients:

For crisp:

- ½ cup + 2 tablespoons quick-cooking rolled oats
- 2 tablespoons unbleached all-purpose flour
- 2 tablespoons brown sugar
- 3 tablespoons non-hydrogenated margarine, melted

For filling:

- ¼ cup brown sugar
- 2 cups fresh or frozen blueberries (do not thaw if frozen)
- ½ tablespoon margarine, melted
- 2 teaspoons cornstarch
- 1 cup grated or chopped apples
- ½ tablespoon lemon juice

Directions:

1. Place rack in the center of the oven.
2. Add all the ingredients for crisp into a bowl and mix until well combined.

3. Add brown sugar and cornstarch into a 6 inch baking dish. Mix well.
4. Add rest of the ingredients for filling and mix well.
5. Sprinkle the crisp over the filling.
6. Bake in a preheated oven at 350° F for about 30 – 45 minutes or until golden brown and crisp on top.
7. Remove from the oven and let it cool for a few minutes before serving. It can be served cold as well

Raspberry Meringue Trifle

Number of servings: 3

Nutritional values per serving:

Calories – 206, Fat – 4 g, Carbohydrate – 38 g, Fiber – 3 g, Protein – 2 g, Sodium – 33 mg, Potassium – 93 mg, Phosphorous – 30 mg, Calcium – NA

Ingredients:

For meringues:

- 1 egg white
- 1/8 teaspoon vanilla extract
- ¼ teaspoon granulated sugar
- 2 tablespoons crushed candy canes

For the raspberry mousse:

- ½ cup frozen raspberries
- 1 teaspoon no sugar added raspberry Jell-O powder
- ½ package fresh raspberries
- 2 tablespoons water
- ¾ cup cool whip

Directions:

1. For meringues: Place a sheet of parchment paper on a small baking sheet.
2. Add egg white into a mixing bowl and beat with an electric hand mixer until fluffy.
3. Add sugar and beat until stiff peaks are formed.
4. Add vanilla and candy canes and fold gently.
5. Spoon onto the prepared baking sheet.

6. Preheat the oven to 350° F. Place the baking sheet in the oven and switch off the oven. Let it remain in the oven for 2 hours. During this time, let the door of the oven remain closed. Open the door only after 2 hours.
7. The meringue would have dried by now. Break into pieces.
8. For the mousse: Add strawberries and water into a small pan. Place over medium heat and cook until slightly soft. Turn off the heat and add into a mixing bowl.
9. Stir in the Jell-O powder. Let it cool completely. Add cool whip and fold gently.
10. To serve: Divide half of each – raspberry mousse followed by meringue and finally fresh raspberries among 3 glasses.
11. Repeat the above step once more.
12. Refrigerate until use.
13. Serve chilled.

Fresh Cranberry Torte

Number of servings: 4

Nutritional values per serving:

Calories – 327, Fat – 19 g, Carbohydrate – 46 g, Fiber – 2 g, Protein – 4 g, Sodium – 38 mg, Potassium – 114 mg, Phosphorous – 26 mg, Calcium – NA

Ingredients:

For crust:

- ¾ cup graham cracker crumbs
- 6 tablespoons Splenda sweetener
- 2 tablespoons chopped, unsalted pecans

For filling:

- ¾ cup ground fresh cranberries
- ½ tablespoon frozen apple juice concentrate, thawed
- 2 cups light Coolwhip whipped topping, thawed
- ½ teaspoon vanilla extract
- ¼ cup unsalted, non-hydrogenated margarine, melted
- 1 egg white
- ½ cup Splenda sweetener

For cranberry glaze:

- 2 tablespoons Splenda sweetener
- ½ tablespoon cornstarch
- 6 tablespoons water
- 2 tablespoons white granulated sugar

- ¼ cup + 2 tablespoons fresh cranberries

Directions:

1. To make the crust: Add all the ingredients for the crust in a bowl and mix well using your hands.
2. Grease transfer into a 6-inch springform pan. Press it well onto the bottom as well as a little on the sides of the pan.
3. Bake in a preheated oven at 375° F for about 30 – 45 minutes or until light brown. Remove from the oven and let it cool.
4. Meanwhile, make the filling as follows: Add berries and Splenda into a bowl and toss well. Let it rest for 5 minutes.
5. Add apple juice concentrate, egg white, and vanilla. Beat with an electric hand mixer on low speed until the froth is formed. Raise the speed to high speed and beat for 5 – 8 minutes or until stiff peaks are formed.
6. Add Cool whip and beat until well combined. Spoon the cranberry filling over the crust. Place in the freezer until frozen.
7. For the glaze: Add all the ingredients for glaze into a saucepan. Place the saucepan over medium heat. Stir frequently until sugar and Splenda dissolves completely.
8. Lower the heat and simmer until the skin of the cranberries begins to crack. Stir occasionally. Turn off the heat and cool completely.
9. Take out the torte from the freezer and place on a serving platter. Spread the glaze over the filling.

10. Cut into 4 equal wedges and serve.

Almond Meringue Cookies

Number of servings: 12

Nutritional values per serving: 2 small cookies

Calories – 37.9, Fat – 0 g, Carbohydrate – 9 g, Fiber – 0 g, Protein – 0.6 g, Sodium – 18 mg, Potassium – 51 mg, Phosphorous – 0.85 mg, Calcium – NA

Ingredients:

- 1 egg white or 2 tablespoons pasteurized egg whites at room temperature
- ¼ teaspoon almond extract
- 3 tablespoons white sugar
- ½ teaspoon cream of tartar
- ¼ teaspoon vanilla extract

Directions:

1. Add egg white and cream of tartar into a bowl. Beat with an electric hand mixer until frothy and twice its original quantity.
2. Add rest of the ingredients and continue beating until stiff peaks form.
3. Line a baking sheet with parchment paper. Drop 1 teaspoon of the batter on the prepared baking sheet. Use another teaspoon to push the batter onto the baking sheet.
4. Bake in a preheated oven at 300° F for about 25 minutes or until they turn crisp.
5. Remove from the oven and cool completely.

6. Transfer into an airtight container.

Sweet Cherry Cobbler

Number of servings: 6

Nutritional values per serving:

Calories – 177, Fat – 2 g, Carbohydrate – 40 g, Fiber – 2 g, Protein – 2 g, Sodium – 103 mg, Potassium – 186 mg, Phosphorous – 65 mg, Calcium – 42 mg

Ingredients:

For the cherry filling:

- 2 ½ cups pitted, halved sweet red cherries
- 1 tablespoon cornstarch
- 1 tablespoon lemon juice
- 1/8 teaspoon almond extract
- ½ teaspoon vanilla extract
- 1/3 cup granulated sugar
- 1/8 teaspoon salt

For topping:

- ½ cup all-purpose flour
- ½ teaspoon baking powder
- 1/8 teaspoon ground cinnamon
- ¼ cup nonfat, cold milk
- ¼ cup sugar
- 1/8 teaspoon salt
- 1 tablespoon unsalted, cold butter, cubed

Directions:

1. For the cherry filling: Add all the ingredients for filling into a saucepan. Place the saucepan over

medium heat. Cook until cherries are soft and the juices get thick.

2. Transfer into a 6-inch baking dish. Do not grease the dish.
3. For the topping: Add all the dry ingredients into a bowl and stir until well combined.
4. Add butter and cut it into the mixture with a fork or pastry cutter until crumbly.
5. Add milk, a little at a time and mix well each time until a soft dough is formed. Use as much milk as required.
6. Drop spoonfuls of the dough at different spots over the filling. Leave some space between the dough.
7. Bake in a preheated oven at 300° F for about 15 minutes or until golden brown on top.
8. Remove from the oven and cool for 20-30 minutes.
9. Serve. Leftovers can be refrigerated for 6-7 days.

Litchi Sorbet

Number of servings: 8

Nutritional values per serving:

Calories – 95, Fat – 0 g, Carbohydrate – 23 g, Fiber – 1 g, Protein – 2 g, Sodium – 15 mg, Potassium – 207 mg, Phosphorous – 36 mg, Calcium – NA

Ingredients:

- 2 cans (14 ounces each) litchis or 2 pounds fresh litchis, peeled, pitted
- 2 pasteurized egg whites
- 4 tablespoons powdered sugar
- Thinly sliced lemon wedges to garnish

Directions:

1. Add litchis and sugar into a blender and blend until smooth.
2. Pass the mixture through a fine wire mesh strainer placed over a bowl. Discard the solids.
3. Pour into a freezer-safe container and place in the freezer for 3 hours.
4. Remove from the freezer and transfer into the food processor bowl process until slush-like inconsistency.
5. With the food processor machine running, drizzle the egg whites through the feeder tube. Process until well combined.
6. Pour the mixture back into the freezer-safe container. Cover and place in the freezer until firm.

7. Transfer into a blender just before serving and blend until slush- like.
8. Scoop into bowls. Garnish with lemon slices and serve.

Apple and Cranberry Cake

Number of servings: 6

Nutritional values per serving:

Calories – 250, Fat – 7 g, Carbohydrate – 50 g, Fiber – 1.6 g, Protein – 3.5 g, Sodium – 183 mg, Potassium – 110.5 mg, Phosphorous – 55 mg, Calcium – NA

Ingredients:

- 3 tablespoons butter
- 1 egg
- ¾ teaspoon baking soda
- 1/3 cup plain yogurt
- 1 apple, cored, peeled, sliced
- ¾ teaspoon ground cinnamon
- 6 tablespoons sugar
- ¾ cup all-purpose flour
- Zest of ½ lemon, grated
- ½ cup cranberries
- ¼ cup brown sugar

Directions:

1. Line a 6-inch baking dish with parchment paper.
2. Add butter and sugar into a bowl and beat with an electric hand mixer until creamy.
3. Add egg and beat well.
4. Add all the dry ingredients into a bowl and stir until well combined.

5. Add dry ingredients into the bowl of butter, a little at a time along with a little zest and a little yogurt each time. Beat well each time.
6. Spoon half the batter into the prepared baking dish.
7. Spread cranberries over the batter. Mix together brown sugar and cinnamon in a bowl and sprinkle half of it over the cranberries.
8. Spoon the remaining batter over the cranberries. Spread it evenly.
9. Place the apple slices over the batter. Sprinkle remaining brown sugar mixture over the apples.
10. Bake in a preheated oven at 350° F for about 45 minutes or until golden brown on top.
11. Remove from the oven and cool for 20-30 minutes.
12. Slice and serve. Leftovers can be refrigerated for 6-7 days.

Raspberry Cheesecake Mousse

Number of servings: 3

Nutritional values per serving:

Calories – 257, Fat – 15 g, Carbohydrate – 29 g, Fiber – 2 g, Protein – 3 g, Sodium – 124 mg, Potassium – 102 mg, Phosphorous – 51 mg, Calcium – NA

Ingredients:

- ½ cup light whipped topping
- 6 tablespoon granular Splenda
- ½ teaspoon vanilla extract
- 4 ounces cream cheese, at room temperature
- ½ teaspoon finely grated lemon zest
- ½ cup fresh or frozen raspberries
- Mint sprigs

Directions:

1. Add cream cheese into a bowl and beat with an electric hand mixer until creamy.
2. Add 4 tablespoons Splenda and beat until it dissolves. Beat in the vanilla and lemon zest.
3. Add whipped topping and fold gently.
4. Set aside a few raspberries to the top and add the remaining into a bowl. Crush with a fork. Add 2 tablespoons Splenda and stir.
5. Add into the cream cheese mixture and fold gently.
6. Divide into 3 small glasses. Refrigerate until use.
7. Top with retained raspberries and mint sprigs and serve.

Conclusion

As we come to the end of the book, I would like to thank you for purchasing it again. I hope this book was helpful in answering your questions on a renal friendly diet.

Both children and adults around the world suffer from kidney disease. It may be an acute or chronic condition, but they all have hope. Taking active steps to improve kidney function and overall health will make a big difference. I hope this cookbook helps you enjoy your meals even while making better renal friendly choices. You will notice the difference as you continue to follow the diet in the long term.

Part 2

Introduction

Heart Health is that every American and over the world citizen should be concerned about. Different heart diseases are one of the main death reasons for both men and women. Moreover, cardiovascular diseases often called as "the silent killer" because it cannot be any warning signs before a heart attack strikes.

Fortunately, heart health is under your control. Surely, there're many factors that cannot be changed, such as age or family history, but you can reduce risk of heart attacks choosing a healthy way of life.

Unfortunately, many people do not use healthy habits for various reasons. Some do not have enough time, some do not have enough knowledge, for some people it's too hard. However, you need to understand that your healthy lifestyle is the best protection against heart diseases, so a healthy way of life is the simplest way to live a long happy life.

Properly formulated diet is one of the easiest and most effective ways to reduce heart diseases attacks. Many people do not know what meals to eat in order to keep the heart and blood vessels healthy. That is why I created this book, which contains delicious, easy, and at the same time useful heart healthy recipes for two that will allow you to eat properly, and also reduce the risk of cardiovascular diseases.

12 Useful tips to minimize risk of heart healthy diseases

Eat heart healthy meals. Make fruit, vegetables, fish, and whole grains the main in your diet.

1. **Limit** sodium, saturated fats and sweets.
2. **Be active.** Try to walk at least 10 000 steps per day.
3. **Control your blood sugar.** Blood glucose should be less than 100 mg/dL
4. **Control your cholesterol.** Total cholesterol should be less than 200 mg/dL
5. **Control your blood pressure.** Try to keep your numbers below 120/80 mm Hg
6. Live smoke-free
7. **Drink more green tea.** It reduces the risk of heart attack.
8. **Reach for vitamin D.** Nearly 75% of heart patients are deficient in Vitamin D.
9. Have an optimistic outlook.
10. **Keep calm.** Try to find 30 minutes per day for relaxation techniques such as deep breathing or meditation.
11. **More muscle – less fat.** Do more physique exercises.

Low Calories Roasted Salmon with Beans & Tomatoes

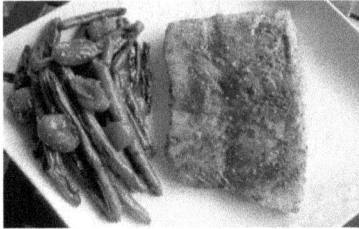

- Prep time: 15 minutes
- Cook time: 20 minutes
- Calories: 304

Ingredients

- 1 large skinless salmon fillet
- 4 clove garlic
- 1 lb. green beans
- 1 pt. grape tomatoes
- 1/2 c. pitted kalamata olives
- 2 tbsp. olive oil
- kosher salt
- Pepper to taste

Directions

1. Preheat oven to 415 F.
2. In the large bowl mix together the garlic, beans, tomatoes, olives, with 1 tablespoon oil and 1/4 teaspoon pepper. Replace to the baking sheet and

roast until the vegetables are tender and beginning to brown.

3. Meanwhile, heat the remaining tablespoon oil in a large skillet over medium heat. Season the salmon with pepper and cook until golden brown and opaque throughout, 4 to 5 minutes per side. Serve with the vegetables.

Fusilli with Broccoli Topping

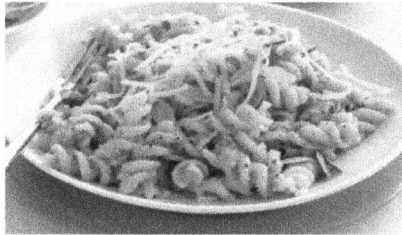

- Prep time: 10 minutes
- Cook time: 15 minutes
- Calories: 340

Ingredients

- 6 oz. fusilli pasta
- 6 oz. frozen broccoli florets
- 1-2 clove garlic
- 1/4 cup fresh basil leaves or 1 tbsp dried basil
- 3 tbsp. olive oil
- 1 tbsp. grated lemon zest
- Parmesan cheese, grated (if desired)

Directions

1. Cook the pasta according to package directions. Reserve 1/2 cup of the cooking liquid, drain the pasta, and return it to the pot.
2. Meanwhile, in a microwave-safe bowl, combine the broccoli, garlic, and 1/2 cup water. Cover and cook on high, stirring once halfway through, until the

broccoli is tender, 5 to 6 minutes. Transfer the mixture (liquid included) to a food processor. Add the basil, oil, zest, and purée until smooth.

3. Toss the pasta with the pesto and 1/4 cup of the reserved liquid. Sprinkle with grated Parmesan cheese if desired.

Delicious Chicken Stir-Fry with Rice

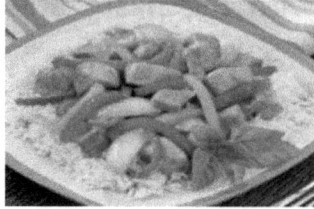

- Prep time: 15 minutes
- Cook time: 30 minutes
- Calories: 432

Ingredients

- 1/2 pound chicken breasts, boneless and skinless
- 1/2 cup brown rice
- 1/4 cup apricot preserves
- 1 tbsp vinegar
- 1 tsp ginger, grated
- A pinch of red pepper flakes
- 3 tbsp olive oil
- 1 medium-sized carrot
- 1/4 pound snow peas

Directions

1. Cook the rice according to package directions.
2. While rice is cooking, in a medium mixing bowl combine apricots, vinegar, grated ginger, pepper flacks and some water. Set aside.

3. Cut lengthwise chicken breasts. Preheat the skillet oven medium-high heat and roast chicken until golden brown, for about 3-5 minutes per side. Transfer to a plate.
4. Add chopped carrots, snow peas and some oil to the skillet and cook for 2-3 minutes, stirring occasionally. Return the chicken fillets to the skillet, pour over the apricot mixture and cook for another 3-4 minutes until vegetables become tender.
5. Serve with rice and enjoy!

Tilapia with Rice, Pineapple and Cucumber

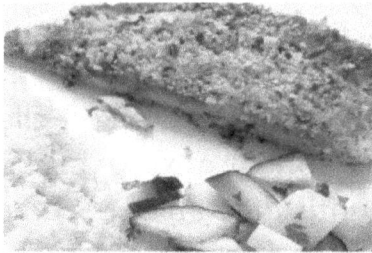

- Prep time: 15 minutes
- Cook time: 20 minutes
- Calories: 370

Ingredients

- 2 medium-sized tilapia fillets
- 1 cup long-grain white rice
- 2 tbsp. fresh lime juice
- 1 tbsp. grated ginger
- 2 tsp. honey
- 2 tbsp. olive oil
- 1 jalapeño pepper, chopped
- 1/2 small pineapple, chopped
- 1 small English cucumber, chopped
- Pepper to taste

Directions

1. Firstly, cook the rice according to package directions.

2. Meanwhile, in a large bowl, whisk together the lime juice, ginger, honey, olive oil and some pepper. Toss with jalapeño, pineapple and cucumber.
3. Heat the remaining tsp oil in a large nonstick skillet over medium heat. Season the tilapia with pepper and cook until golden brown and cooked through, 1 to 3 minutes per side. Serve the fish with the rice and vegetable mixture.

Delicious Sugar Snap Peas and Radish Salad

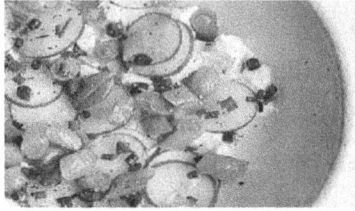

- Prep time: 10 minutes
- Cook time: 10 minutes
- Calories: 135

Ingredients

- 1 pound sugar snap peas
- 12 small radishes
- 1/2 medium ripe avocado
- 2 tbsp. apple-cider vinegar
- 1 tbsp. fresh lemon juice
- 1/2 tsp. Dijon mustard
- 1/2 tsp. salt
- 1/2 tsp. Freshly ground pepper
- 1/4 tsp. ground coriander
- 3 tbsp olive oil

Directions

1. In a large bowl, combine sugar snap peas and radishes. Set aside.
2. In a blender or the bowl of a food processor, combine avocado, vinegar, lemon juice, mustard,

salt, pepper, and coriander. Gradually add oil, blending until mixture is a smooth purée. If needed add couple tbsp water.

3. Toss salad with dressing to coat and serve immediately.

Heart Healthy Bean Burrito Bowl

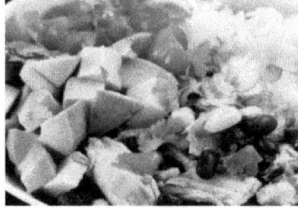

- Prep time: 20 minutes
- Cook time: 25 minutes
- Calories: 312

Ingredients

- 1 cup cooked brown rice
- 1 small avocado
- 1/2 can black beans
- 2 tbsp fresh lime juice
- 2 tbsp olive oil
- 1/2 tsp. ground cumin
- 1/4 head romaine lettuce
- 1 tbsp dried cilantro
- 5 cherry tomatoes, cut
- 1/2 small red onion
- 2 tbsp low-fat sour cream
- Tortilla chips, lime wedges for dressing
- Hot sauce to taste

Directions

1. In a small mixing bowl, whisk together the lime juice, oil, and cumin.
2. Divide the rice and beans among serving bowls. Top with the lettuce, cilantro, tomatoes, and avocado.
3. Sprinkle with the red onion, then drizzle with the dressing. Serve with sour cream, tortilla chips, lime wedges, and hot sauce, if desired.

Chickpea and Red Pepper Soup with Quinoa

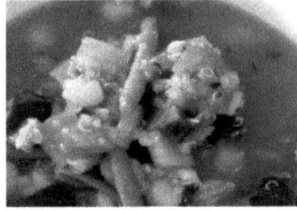

- Prep time: 20 minutes
- Cook time: 25 minutes
- Calories: 384

Ingredients

- 1/4 cup uncooked quinoa
- 2 tbsp olive oil
- 1 small onion, chopped
- 1 small carrot, chopped
- 1 stalk celery, chopped
- 2 garlic cloves, minced
- 1 tsp smoked paprika
- A pinch of salt and pepper
- 1 medium yellow bell pepper
- 1 medium red bell pepper
- 1 can low-sodium chickpeas
- 1 cup low-sodium vegetable broth
- 1 tbsp red wine vinegar
- Chopped fresh parsley for garnish

Directions

1. Cook the quinoa according to package directions.
2. While cooking heat the oil in a Dutch oven or large heavy-bottomed pot. Add the onion, carrot, and celery and cook, covered, stirring occasionally, for 6 minutes.
3. Then, add garlic, paprika, season with salt and pepper and cook, stirring, for 1 minute. Add bell peppers and cook for another 5 minutes.
4. Add the chickpeas, broth, and 1 cup water and bring to a boil. Reduce heat and simmer until the vegetables are tender, 5 to 8 minutes. Stir in the vinegar and cooked quinoa. Serve topped with parsley, if desired.

Sweet and Spicy Glazed Salmon with Delicious Rice

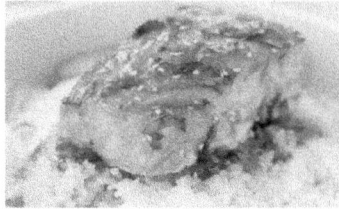

- Prep time: 15 minutes
- Cook time: 25 minutes
- Calories: 498

Ingredients

- 2 salmon fillets
- 1/2 cup long-grain white rice
- 5 tbsp sliced almonds
- 1 small orange
- 1/4 cup hot pepper jelly
- A pinch of salt and pepper to taste
- Freshly chopped parsley

Directions

1. Heat oven to 390 F. Cook the rice according to package directions.
2. While rice cooking, spread the almonds on a baking sheet and roast until light golden brown, for 5 minutes. Then transfer to a bowl. Heat broiler. Line

a broiler-proof rimmed baking sheet with nonstick foil.

3. Squeeze the juice from half an orange into a small bowl and get 2 tablespoons juice. Add the jelly and whisk to combine. Place the salmon on the baking sheet, season with 1/2 teaspoon each salt and pepper, and roast for 5 minutes. Spoon half the jelly mixture over the salmon and broil until the salmon is opaque throughout, 2 to 5 minutes more.

4. Cut remain half of the orange into 1/2-inch pieces. Fold the oranges, almonds, and parsley into the rice. Serve with the salmon and the remaining jelly mixture.

Black Bean and Avocado Salsa

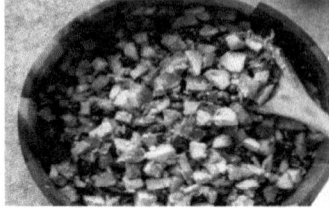

- Prep time: 10 minutes
- Cook time: 15 minutes
- Calories: 143

Ingredients

- 1/2 can black beans
- 1 garlic clove, minced
- 1 jalapeño pepper
- 1 small onion, chopped
- Salt and pepper to taste
- 2 scallions
- 2 tbsp. fresh lime juice
- 1 tbsp. olive oil
- 1 medium-sized avocado
- 1 tsp dried cilantro

Directions

1. In a large bowl, combine chopped jalapeño, garlic, onion, and season with salt and pepper.
2. Add beans, scallions, lime juice, and oil and toss to combine. Fold in the avocado and cilantro.

3. Serve and enjoy!

Quinoa Bowl with Red Pepper, Green Beans, and Red Onion

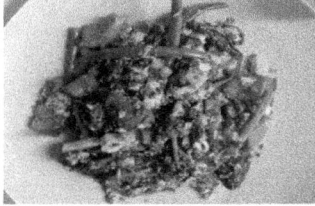

- Prep time: 10 minutes
- Cook time: 15 minutes
- Calories: 154

Ingredients

- 1/2 cup uncooked quinoa
- 1/4 tsp salt
- 1/4 tsp pepper
- 1 jarred roasted red pepper
- 2 oz green beans
- 1 small red onion, chopped
- 1 tbsp olive oil
- 2 tsp red wine vinegar

Directions

1. Place quinoa in a medium saucepan and pour with 2 cups water. Bring to a boil, add some salt, then reduce heat and simmer, covered, until all the liquid has absorbed, nearly 10 minutes.

2. While cooking, in a large bowl, whisk together oil and vinegar, season with salt and pepper, stir to combine. Add red peppers, beans, and onion and toss to combine. Add the prepared quinoa mix evenly. Serve.

Avocados with Creamy Crab Salad

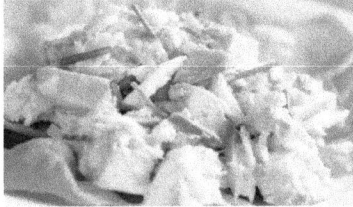

- Prep time: 3 minutes
- Cook time: 5 minutes
- Calories: 519

Ingredients

- 3 firm ripped avocados
- 1 tbsp grated lemon zest
- 4 tbsp fresh lemon juice
- 1 pound lump crab meat
- 1/4 cup radishes, diced
- 4 tbsp light mayonnaise
- 1 tsp dried basil

Directions

1. Cut 2 avocados in half. Chop remaining avocado in 1/2-inch dice. Sprinkle 2 tablespoons of the lemon juice over halved and diced avocados.
2. In large bowl combine diced avocado, lemon zest, the remaining 2 tablespoons lemon juice, crab meat, radishes, mayonnaise, and basil, tossing lightly.

3. Spoon mixture into the cut halves of avocado.
4. Serve with grilled or toasted pita bread if desired.

Horseradish Salmon Cakes

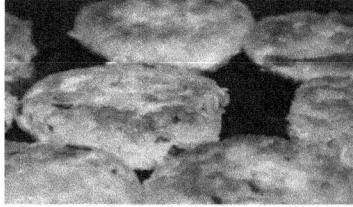

- Prep time: 15 minutes
- Cook time: 20 minutes
- Calories: 301

Ingredients

- 2 medium-sized salmon fillets
- 1 tbsp prepared horseradish
- 1 tbsp Dijon mustard
- 5 tbsp Panko bread crumbs
- 2 tbsp olive oil
- 2 tbsp fat-less Greek yogurt
- 1 tbsp fresh lemon juice
- 1 small English cucumber
- A bunch watercress
- A pinch of salt and pepper to taste

Directions

1. In a food processor blend the salmon, horseradish, mustard, salt, and pepper until coarsely chopped. Stir in bread crumbs and form the mixture into 8 patties.

131

2. Heat 1 tablespoon oil in a large nonstick skillet over medium heat. Cook the patties until brown, 2 minutes per side.
3. In a large bowl, whisk together the yogurt, lemon juice, remaining oil. Season with salt and pepper. Add the cucumbers and toss to coat; fold in the watercress. Serve with the patties.

Balsamic Chicken with Apple, Lentil, and Spinach Salad

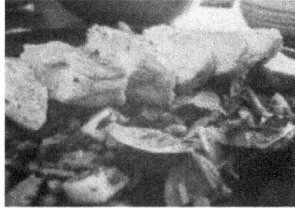

- Prep time: 15 minutes
- Cook time: 20 minutes
- Calories: 387

Ingredients

- 1 large chicken breast, boneless and skinless
- 1 scallions
- 1 small green apple
- 1 stalk celery
- 1 tbsp fresh lemon juice
- 1/2 can lentils
- 1 cup baby spinach
- 1/4 cup fresh flat-leaf parsley
- 3 tbsp olive oil
- A pinch of salt and pepper to taste
- 2 tbsp balsamic vinegar

Directions

1. Heat 1 tablespoon oil in a large skillet over medium heat. Season the chicken with salt and pepper and

cook until golden brown, nearly 6-7 minutes each side. Remove from heat and add the vinegar. Turn the chicken to coat.

2. While cooking, in a large bowl, place scallions, apple, celery, lemon juice, 1 tablespoon oil, season with salt and pepper. Fold in the lentils, spinach and parsley (if desired) and serve with the chicken.

Heart Healthy Minestrone Soup

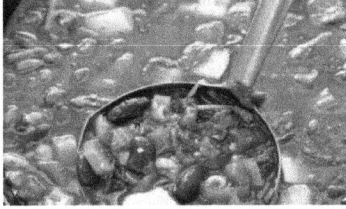

- Prep time: 10 minutes
- Cook time: 20 minutes
- Calories: 286

Ingredients

- 1/2 pound asparagus, trimmed and cut into 1-inch pieces
- 1/2 can white beans, rinsed
- 2 tbsp olive oil
- 1 stalk celery, chopped
- 1 leek (white and light green parts only), finely chopped
- 1 small onion, chopped
- 2 medium-sized potatoes, cut in 1/2-inch pieces
- 3 sprigs fresh thyme
- 3 oz. sugar snap peas, halved
- Some freshly chopped dill for serving
- A pinch of salt and pepper to taste

Directions

1. Heat oil in a Dutch oven on medium. Add celery, leeks, onion, season with salt and pepper and cook, covered, stirring occasionally, until tender.
2. Add potatoes, thyme, and 6 cups water and bring to a boil, then simmer 8 minutes. Add asparagus and simmer 2 minutes.
3. Add sugar snap peas and beans and simmer until vegetables are just tender, 3 to 4 minutes more. Discard thyme sprigs. Sprinkle soup with dill and serve.

Delicious Tortilla Fish Sticks with Purple Cabbage Slaw

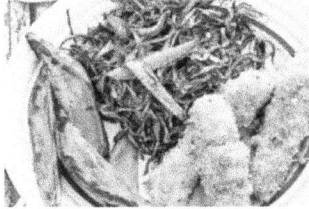

- Prep time: 5 minutes
- Cook time: 25 minutes
- Calories: 376

Ingredients

- 1 pound tilapia fillets
- 1/2 small red cabbage, cored and finely chopped
- 1 small orange
- 3 tbsp fresh lime juice
- 1 tsp sugar
- 5 tbsp sour cream
- 1 medium-sized carrot, grated
- 1 small red onion, chopped
- 2 cups tortilla chips, crushed
- 1 tsp dried cilantro
- 1/4 tsp salt
- 1/4 tsp pepper

Directions

1. Heat oven to 425°F. Take the large bowl and grate 1 tsp zest from orange into it. Squeeze in juice (about 1/3 cup). Whisk in lime juice, add sugar, salt and pepper to taste, whisk in sour cream.
2. Transfer 1/2 cup mixture to a shallow bowl. Add carrots, onion, and cabbage to the large bowl and let sit.
3. Meanwhile, line a rimmed baking sheet with foil. Cut tilapia into large chunks. Dip fish in reserved sour cream mixture and then in crushed chips, pressing gently to help them adhere.
4. Transfer fish chunks to the baking sheet and cook until light golden brown for about 8-10 minutes. Fold cilantro into slaw and serve with fish.

Spaghetti Squash and Chickpea Sauté

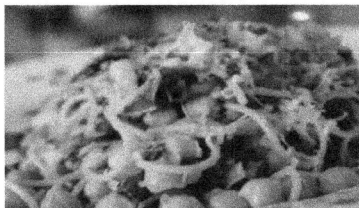

- Prep time: 5 minutes
- Cook time: 15 minutes
- Calories: 289

Ingredients

- 1 pound spaghetti squash
- 1 small red onion, finely chopped
- 3 tbsp fresh lemon juice
- 2 tbsp olive oil
- 1 garlic clove, minced
- 1/2 can chickpeas, rinsed
- 1/2 cup fresh flat-leaf parsley, chopped
- 2 oz crumbled feta
- Ground black pepper to taste

Directions

1. Prepare spaghetti squash and halve with large knife. Place them on a large paper sheet and microwave on high for 5-7 minutes until tender. Transfer cooked spaghetti to a large bowl.

2. Meanwhile, in a small mixing bowl toss onion, lemon juice and season with salt and pepper.
3. Sprinkle a non-stick skillet with 1 tbsp olive oil and toss minced garlic. Cook until golden brown. Add rinsed chickpeas and cook for couple minutes. Add spaghetti squash and 1 tablespoon olive oil.
4. Top with crumbled feta and serve.

Cod Fillets with Potatoes and Bacon

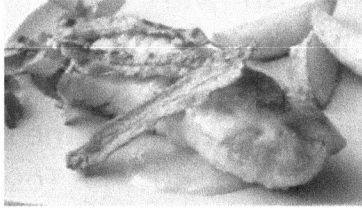

- Prep time: 15 minutes
- Cook time: 15 minutes
- Calories: 415

Ingredients

- 2 large cod fillets (1 inch thick)
- 2 slices bacon, cut into 1/2-inch pieces
- 1/2 pound small potatoes, halved
- 1 medium red onion cut into 1/2 inch lengthwise
- 1 tbsp. mayonnaise
- 1 tbsp. Dijon mustard
- 5 tbsp panko bread crumbs
- 1 tbsp olive oil
- 1 tbsp Thyme leaves
- Salt and black pepper

Directions

1. Preheat the oven to 450 F. Place potatoes and onions in the center of a baking sheet and place bacon on top. Roast for 10 minutes.

2. While potatoes are cooking, in a medium mixing bowl combine mayonnaise and mustard. In another bowl, combine Panko with oil, then sprinkle with thyme. Season fish with salt and pepper, then spread with mayonnaise mixture and sprinkle with Panko.
3. Remove the baking sheet from the oven and reduce oven temperature to 400 F. Toss potatoes and onion mixture together, then spread in an even layer, arranging potatoes cut side down.
4. Nestle fish pieces among vegetables and roast until fish is tender and lightly golden, for about 10-12 minutes.

Slow Cooker Pork with Spinach Rice

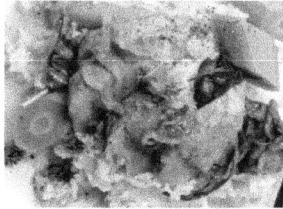

- Prep time: 15 minutes
- Cook time: 2 hours
- Calories: 475

Ingredients

- 1/2 pound pork tenderloin
- 1/2 cup long-grain white rice
- 1 small green apple
- 1 small onion
- 1 tbsp flour
- 1 cup baby spinach
- 2 large carrots (about 1/2 pound), cut into 2-inch pieces
- 2 tbsp Dijon mustard
- 2 tbsp honey
- 1 tbsp low-sodium soy sauce
- 4 sprigs fresh thyme, plus extra leaves for serving
- Salt and pepper to taste

Directions

1. Chop apple and onion and add to a slow cooker bowl. Toss with the flour and then add carrots.
2. In another mixing bowl combine mustard, honey and soy sauce. Cut the pork into 2 pieces and place to a slow cooker. Pour with the mustard mixture and mix to combine. Sprinkle with salt and pepper and add some thyme on top.
3. Secure the lid and cook until carrots are tender, about 2 hours.
4. Meanwhile, cook rice according the package directions.
5. Open the lid and discard the thyme. Transfer the meat to the cutting board and slice it. Add baby spinach to the slow cooker and stir to combine well. Serve sliced pork with rice and veggies, sprinkle with some fresh dill or cilantro if desired.

Amazing Pork and Vegetable Stir-Fry

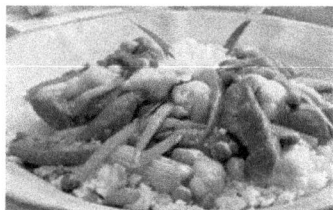

- Prep time: 30 minutes
- Cook time: 30 minutes
- Calories: 359

Ingredients

- 1/2 cup long-grain white rice
- 1/2 pound pork
- 2 tbsp hoisin sauce
- 1 tbsp fresh lime juice
- 2 tbsp canola oil
- 1 medium carrot, sliced
- 1 small red bell pepper, sliced
- A pinch of salt and pepper
- 1/2 cup bean sprouts

Directions

1. Cook the rice according to package directions.
2. In a small mixing bowl, combine hoisin sauce, lime juice and 1 tablespoon water. Mix well and set aside.

3. On a large skillet add 1 tablespoon oil and heat over medium heat. Add the carrots and bell pepper and cook, stirring frequently, until tender, nearly 5 minutes. Transfer to a bowl.
4. Return the skillet to the stove, add another tablespoon of oil. Season the pork with salt and pepper and fry on a skillet, flipping couple times, Pour in the hoisin mixture and cook for 1 minute.
5. Return the vegetables to the skillet, add the bean sprouts (if using) and cook, tossing, until heated through, about 2 minutes. Serve over the rice and enjoy.

Classic Beef & Broccoli

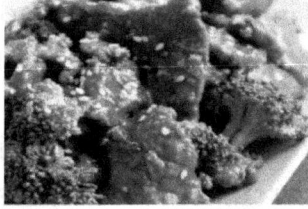

- Prep time: 25 minutes
- Cook time: 25 minutes
- Calories: 412

Ingredients

- 1/2 pound pork steak, halved lengthwise, then very thinly sliced crosswise
- 1 cup broccoli, cut into small florets
- 2 tbsp low-sodium soy sauce
- 4 tsp rice vinegar
- 2 cloves garlic, minced
- 1 tbsp brown sugar
- 1 tsp grated fresh ginger
- 1 tsp cornstarch
- 1 tbsp canola oil
- 1 small red chili, thinly sliced
- 2 scallions, thinly sliced

Directions

1. In a mixing bowl combine soy sauce and vinegar, add minced garlic. Add the meat and set aside for 5-10 minutes.
2. Place broccoli in a large skillet, add some water and simmer until nearly tender and bright green. Transfer to a plate.
3. Meanwhile, in another bowl mix together sugar, ginger, cornstarch, some soy sauce and vinegar, couple tbsp water.
4. Add the oil to a skillet and heat. Add beef in one layer and cook for 1-2 minutes. Add the sauce and simmer until meat will be tender. Add the broccoli and scallions and toss to combine.
5. Serve with or without rice.

Cod with Green Beans

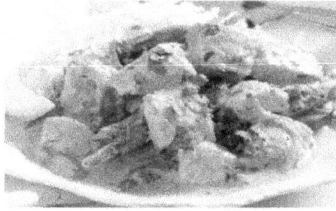

- Prep time: 5 minutes
- Cook time: 20 minutes
- Calories: 240

Ingredients

- 2 cod fillets
- 1/2 pound green beans
- 2 tbsp olive oil
- 1/4 cup Parmesan, grated
- 2 tbsp basil pesto
- Salt and pepper to taste

Directions

1. Preheat the oven to 420 F. Place beans on a large baking sheet, sprinkle with olive oil, season with salt and pepper, sprinkle with grated Parmesan. Roast until golden for about 10 minutes.
2. While cooking, preheat the large skillet with 1 tbsp oil. Season the cod with salt and pepper and fry fish from both sides until golden for about 2-4 minutes.

3. Spoon the pesto over the cod and serve with the beans.

Tilapia with Zoodles

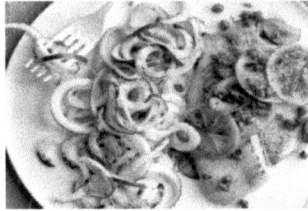

- Prep time: 10 minutes
- Cook time: 20 minutes
- Calories: 287

Ingredients

- 1 medium-sized zucchini, spiralized
- 2 medium tilapia fillets
- 3 tbsp olive oil
- 1/2 lemon, sliced
- 2 garlic cloves, chopped
- 1 tbsp capers (if desired)
- Freshly chopped parsley for garnish

Directions

1. Preheat the oven to 450 F. Take a baking sheet and place spiralized zucchini. Sprinkle with the olive oil and season with salt and pepper. Cook until tender and lightly golden for about 8-10 minutes.

2. While cooking, preheat the large skillet with 1 tablespoon olive oil on a medium heat. Season tilapia fillets with salt and pepper from both sides and fry for 3-5 minutes, until ready. Transfer to a plate.
3. Add 1 tbsp olive oil, then lemon, garlic, capers, and cook for couple minutes, stirring occasionally, for 2-4 minutes.
4. Serve fish, zoodles and lemon mixture, garnish with freshly chopped parsley and enjoy.

Chicken Fillets Marinated in Yogurt

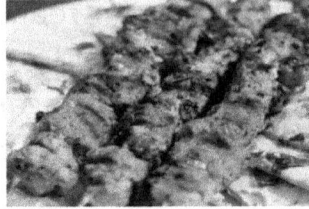

- Prep time: 30 minutes
- Cook time: 30 minutes
- Calories: 398

Ingredients

- 1 pound chicken breasts, boneless and skinless, cubed into 2-inch pieces
- 1/2 cup non-fat yogurt
- 2 garlic cloves, minced
- 1 tbsp grated ginger
- 1/2 tsp curry powder
- 1 tbsp lemon zest, grated
- 2 tbsp lemon juice
- 1 large bell pepper cut into 2-inch pieces
- 1 tbsp oil
- Salt and pepper to taste

Directions

1. In a large mixing bowl, combine the yogurt, garlic, ginger, curry powder, lemon zest, 2 tablespoons lemon juice. Season with salt and pepper and stir to

combine. Add chicken cubes and set aside for 15 minutes.
2. Preheat your grill to medium-high. Thread the chicken and peppers onto skewers. Lightly oil the grill and cook the kebabs, turning couple times, until cooked through, 8 to 10 minutes.
3. Serve with rice, couscous or vegetables.

Spicy Lamb with Veggies

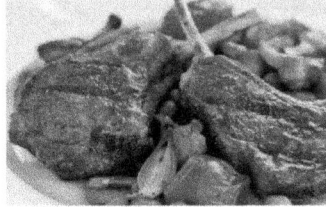

- Prep time: 20 minutes
- Cook time: 20 minutes
- Calories: 341

Ingredients

- 4 small lamb chops
- 2 medium-sized carrots
- 5 large radishes
- 3 tbsp olive oil
- 2 tbsp red wine vinegar
- 1/2 tsp honey
- 1/2 tsp ground cumin
- A pinch of salt and pepper

Directions

1. In a medium mixing bowl combine oil, vinegar, honey, cumin, season salt and pepper, and whisk to combine well. Set aside.
2. Preheat the skillet over medium-high heat. Sprinkle with tbsp of olive oil. Season the lamb chops with

salt and pepper and cook on skillet to desired doneness - 4-6 minutes from each side.

3. While frying, use a vegetable peeler to make thin carrot strips and thin radish slices. Transfer veggies to a large bowl and cover with vinegar mixture. Combine well and serve with cooked lamb chops.

Pork Medallions with Herbs

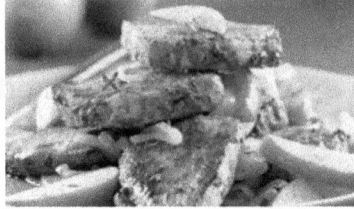

- Prep time: 20 minutes
- Cook time: 35 minutes
- Calories: 276

Ingredients

- 1 pound pork tenderloin
- 2 medium-sized carrots
- 1/2 pound asparagus
- 2 tbsp olive oil
- 1/2 cup freshly chopped parsley
- 1/2 tsp dried rosemary
- 1 package baby greens and herbs
- A pinch of salt and pepper

Directions

1. In a bowl combine chopped parsley and rosemary. Rub this mixture over the tenderloin and set aside.
2. Boil carrots for 5 minutes, chill. Do the same with asparagus for 3 minutes, until bright green and crisp.
3. Preheat oven to 380 F.

4. Cover the pork tenderloin with salt and pepper, preheat the ovenproof skillet and cook meat for 5-8 minutes until brown. Transfer to an oven and cook until ready and tender.
5. Meanwhile, cut carrots and asparagus into 2-inch-long sticks. Transfer to a large bowl, add baby greens, and remaining parsley. Season with salt and pepper and add remaining tablespoon oil. Add balsamic vinegar and stir to combine. Divide salad among serving plates.
6. Slice pork tenderloin and serve on the top of the salads.

How to make your own sodium-substitute seasonings

SPICY MIX
What you will need
1/4 teaspoon curry powder
2 tablespoons dried savory, crumbled
1 tablespoon dry mustard
1/4 teaspoon ground cumin
1/3 teaspoon garlic powder
1/3 teaspoon freshly ground white pepper
3 teaspoons onion powder

How to prepare
1. Mix all the ingredients in a small bowl and blend well.
2. SPOON THE BLENDED MIX INTO A SHAKER AND STORE IN A COOL, DARK PLACE.

HERB SEASONING
What you will need
Pinch freshly ground pepper
2 tablespoons dried basil leaves or dill weed, crumbled
2 tablespoons onion powder
1 teaspoon celery seed
1/4 dried oregano leaves crumbled

How to prepare
1. MIX ALL THE INGREDIENTS IN A SMALL BOWL AND BLEND WELL.

158

2. Spoon the blended mix into a shaker and store in a cool, dark place.

A standard menu for breakfast, lunch, dinner and snacks

If you are confused about how to formulate a menu or what to include in your meals, then this subheading will help you decided how to eat low-sodium diets throughout the day.

What to eat for breakfast

- Milk
- Fresh fruit
- LOW-SODIUM CEREAL, HOT OR COLD

What to eat for lunch

- Vanilla wafers
- Applesauce
- Raw carrot sticks
- LEAN ROAST TURKEY ON WHOLE WHEAT BREAD WITH LOW-SODIUM MUSTARD

What to snack on

- Yoghurt
- Fruits
- Almonds or walnuts
- RAISINS

What to eat for dinner

- Fresh melon

- Grilled chicken
- Tossed salad and low-sodium dressing
- Boiled potatoes
- STEAMED FRESH VEGETABLES

Tips to help you cut down on sodium intake

1. Always select to eat foods that are low in salt. In case you frequent the grocery, it is best to read food labels before buying them. Low sodium is defined as 140mg of sodium per serving. Furthermore, since salt substitutes are sometimes gotten from potassium, potassium is a good alternative except you are on a low potassium diet.
2. Cooking is creativity, so be creative. You can season your foods with spices, garlic, herbs, ginger, vinegar, pepper and lemon.
3. Cook your own meals. This is in fact the best way to control your salt intake.
4. Avoid using softened water for drinking and cooking; it contains added salt.
5. RUN FROM MEDICATIONS THAT CONTAIN SODIUM SUCH AS BROMO SELTZER AND ALKA SELTZER.

Selecting What To Eat

Dairy Products

High-Sodium

- Cottage cheese
- Buttermilk
- REGULAR AND PROCESSED SAUCES, CHEESE AND CHEESE SPREADS

Low-Sodium

Low-sodium cheeses, ricotta cheese, cream cheese and mozzarella

Meats, Poultry, Fish, Eggs, Nuts and Legumes

High-Sodium Foods

- Salted nuts
- Smoked, cured, salted or canned fish, meat, or poultry including cold cuts, frankfurters, sardines, bacon, sausage, caviar and anchovies
- Canned entrees, such as ravioli, spam and chili
- Beans canned with added salt
- FROZEN BREADED MEATS AND DINNERS, SUCH AS PIZZA AND BURRITOS

Low-Sodium

- Drained, water or oil packed canned fish or poultry
- Any frozen or fresh beef, pork, lamb, poultry and fish

- Low-sodium peanut butter
- Eggs and egg substitutes
- Low-sodium canned fish
- UN-CANNED, DRY PEAS AND BEANS

Breads, Grains and Cereals

High-Sodium
- Pizza, croutons and salted crackers
- Bread and rolls with salted tops
- Prepackaged, process mixes for rice, potatoes and pasta
- QUICK BREADS, BISCUIT, PANCAKE AND SELF-RISING FLOUR

Low-Sodium
- Low-sodium corn and flour tortillas and noodles
- Unsalted popcorn, pretzels and chips
- Breads, bagels and rolls (no salted tops)
- Muffins and ready-to-eat cereals
- ALL PASTA AND RICE (BUT AVOID ADDING SALT WHEN COOKING)

Soups
- High-Sodium
- Cup of noodles and seasoned ramen mixes
- REGULAR CANNED AND DEHYDRATED SOUP, BOUILLON AND BROTH

Low-Sodium
- Homemade soups (don't add salt)

- LOW-SODIUM CANNED AND DEHYDRATED SOUPS, BOUILLON AND BROTH

Fruits and Vegetables

High-Sodium

- Commercially prepared pasta and tomato sauces and salsa
- Vegetables made with ham, unsalted pork or bacon
- Olives, sauerkraut, pickles and other pickled vegetables
- REGULAR CANNED VEGETABLES AND VEGETABLE JUICES

Low-Sodium

- Dried nuts
- Low-sodium canned vegetables, sauces and juices (rinse canned vegetables to remove some sodium)
- Most fresh, frozen and canned fruit and vegetables
- Fresh fruits like bananas, apples and oranges
- Fresh vegetables like spinach, carrots and broccoli
- FROZEN FRENCH FRIES, FRESH TOMATOES AND INSTANT MASHED TOMATOES

Fats, Desserts and Sweets

Low-Sodium

- Instant cake and pudding
- Seasoning salt, soy sauce, other available sauces and marinades
- Salted margarine or butter

- Ketchup, mustard
- REGULAR SALAD DRESSING WITH BACON BITS AND BOTTLED SALAD DRESSINGS

Low-Sodium
- All deserts prepared without salt
- Unsalted butter or margarine, vinegar
- Mayonnaise
- Low sodium sauces, vegetable oils and salad dressings

3

Recipes for Preparing Mouth-Watering Diets That Are Completely Low In Sodium

Split Pea Soup with Ham

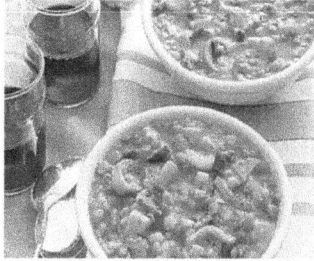

This dish was actually introduced to the U.S. by early English settlers. It has become a favorite across the nation. In lieu of salt, smoked paprika has been selected for a tasty, smoky flavor. This recipe will yield 7 servings.

What you will need
1 leek
1 cup sliced celery
1/2 teaspoon Spanish smoked paprika
1 bay leaf
1/4 teaspoon salt
1/2 teaspoon freshly ground black pepper
4 ounces ham, cut into 1/2-inch cubes
1/2 teaspoon dried tarragon
1 cup lower-sodium chicken broth
2 bacon slices, cut crosswise into 1/4-inch slices
1 pound green split peas
1 1/2 cup chopped carrot

7 cups water

1 teaspoon dried thyme

How to prepare

1. Sort, wash, and drain spilt peas. Take out outer leaves, roots, and tops from leeks, leaving 1/2-inch of dark leaves. Slice leek in half lengthwise, cut each half into thin slices, and rinse well with cold water.

2. In a large saucepan, cook bacon over medium-high heat until crisp. Add celery, onion, oil, carrot, and leek. Cook for 8 minutes over medium heat, stirring occasionally.

3. Add split peas and allow for an additional 1 minute, constantly stirring. Next, add 7 cups water, lower sodium chicken broth, dried thyme, dried tarragon, freshly ground black pepper, salt, and bay leaf. Let to boil over medium-low heat for 45 minutes, or until split peas become tender.

4. THROW AWAY BAY LEAF. STIR IN SMOKED PAPRIKA AND HAM, AND LET TO SIMMER FOR 2 MINUTES. ONCE COOL, SERVE IMMEDIATELY.

Jambalaya

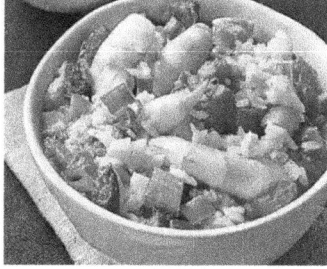

This dish is spicy and tasty with a great feel of onion, bell pepper and celery. This recipe will yield 6 servings.

What you will need

1 1/2 cup chopped onion

2 cups cooked whole-grain rice

2 cups chicken broth

5 garlic cloves, minced

1 1/2 teaspoons canola oil

1 cup chopped green bell pepper

6 ounces Andouille sausage chopped

1/4 teaspoon salt

3 1/2 tablespoons sliced green onions

1 can unsalted diced tomatoes, undrained (14.5-ounces)

12 ounces large shrimp, peeled

1/2 cup chopped celery

How to prepare

1. Heat a large skillet over medium-high heat. Swirl oil in pan to coat. Add sausage and sauté for 3 minutes or until brown.
2. Reduce heat to medium and add bell pepper, onion, and celery. Let to cook for7 minutes, occasionally stirring. Then add garlic, stirring constantly for 1 minute.
3. Stir in rice and red pepper, stirring for 1 minute. Stir in tomatoes, salt, and broth; cover, reduce heat, and simmer for 8 minutes, or until liquid is almost absorbed.
4. Nestle shrimp into rice mixture. Cover and simmer for 6 minutes, or until shrimp are almost done. Uncover and cook for additional 4 minutes, or until shrimp are done.
5. PUT DOWN FROM HEAT AND SPREAD TOP WITH GREEN ONIONS.

Banana Bread with Chocolate Glaze

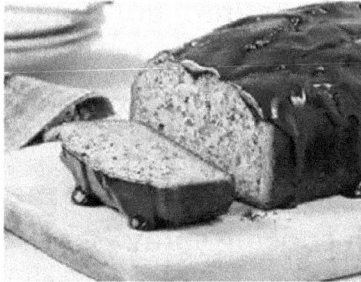

This dish is so irresistible, with sweet chocolate smell and look. With a total time of 1 hour 50 minutes, you'll get 16 servings from this bread.

What you will need
Cooking spray
1 teaspoon baking soda
1/2 teaspoon salt
2 ounces finely chopped semisweet chocolate
1 cup sugar
1 1/2 cups mashed ripe banana (or 3 bananas)
1/4 cup reduced-fat sour cream
1/4 cup fat-free milk
2 1/2 teaspoons half-and-half
9 ounces all-purpose flour, unbleached
2 large egg whites
  How to prepare
1. Preheat oven to 350 degrees F.

2. Mix butter and sugar in a bowl and beat with a mixer until well blended. Add milk, banana, sour cream, and egg whites.
3. Lightly spoon flour into dry measuring cups; level with knife. Mix baking soda, flour, and salt, whisk together. Then add flour mixture to banana mixture and blend (do not overheat).
4. Spoon batter into a 9 by 5-inch metal loaf pan that is coated with cooking spray.
5. Bake for about 1 hour or until a wooden pick inserted in the center comes out clean. Leave to cool in the pan for 10 minutes; remove from pan and cool on a wire rack.
6. Next, place chocolate and half-and-half in a microwave-safe bowl and microwave at high for a minute or until chocolate melts. Ensure you are stirring every 20 seconds.
7. COOL A BIT AND DRIZZLE OVER BREAD.

Broccoli Cheddar Soup

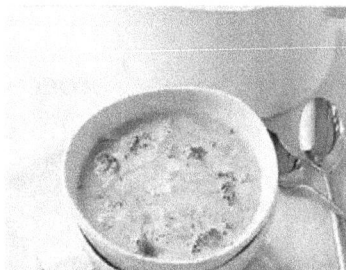

This is a hearty and satisfying soup that gets its rich creaminess from potatoes. It takes a total cook time f 30 minutes and yields a total of 6 servings.

What you will need
3 tablespoons butter, unsalted
4 cups cubed peeled baking potato
1/4 teaspoon salt
1/3 cup carrot, chopped
1 minced garlic clove
4 ounces reduced fat sharp cheddar cheese, shredded
2 cups water, divided and 2 teaspoons of water
2 cups 1% low-fat milk
51/2 cups chopped fresh broccoli florets, divide
1 cup chopped onion
3 cups fat free, low-sodium chicken broth
How to prepare
1. In a large saucepan, place potato and 1/4 teaspoon salt and add water to cover.

2. Boil over reduced heat and simmer for 10 minutes or until tender. Drain afterward.
3. Over medium heat, melt butter in a large Dutch oven. Then sauté carrot, garlic and onion for 5 minutes or until tender.
4. Add 2 cups water, 4 cups broccoli, and bring to simmer. Allow to cook for 10 minutes before stirring in potatoes.
5. Mix 2 teaspoons water and 1 cup broccoli in a microwave-safe bowl. Cover and allow to microwave at high heat for 1 minute or until bright green. Drain afterwards.
6. Process the mix in Dutch oven using a hand-held immersion blender until smooth.
7. Add cheese and milk, and cook over low heat for 2 minutes, stirring until cheese melts and soup is smooth.
8. STIR IN THE STEAMED BROCCOLI AND LADLE INTO INDIVIDUAL BOWLS.

Butter Crunch Lemon Bars

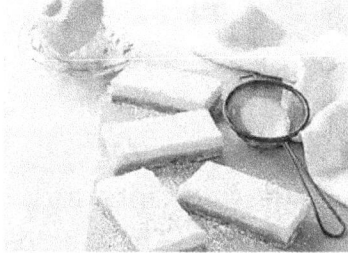

If you are looking for low-sodium, buttery, crunchy dish with lemon feeling then you should consider this recipe. If you don't really like lemons, fresh orange juice and grated orange rind is a great substitute.

What you will need
1 cup 4.5 ounces all-purpose flour
1/4 teaspoon ground mace
Crust
1/4 cup packed dark brown sugar
1/3 cup softened butter
Cooking spray
1 cup sugar, granulated
2 large eggs
1 tablespoon grated lemon rand
1 large egg white
3 tablespoons fresh lemon juice
1 cup 1% low-fat cottage cheese
2 teaspoons all-purpose flour

Powdered sugar (if you wish)

How to prepare
1. Preheat oven to 250 degrees F.
2. Prepare crust by placing crust, 1/3 cup butter, dark brown sugar and 1/4 teaspoon salt in a bowl, and beat with a mixer until smooth.
3. Lightly spoon 1 cup flour into a dry measuring cup, using a knife to level. Then add flour to butter mixture and beat until well blended.
4. Press crust into the bottom of an 8-inch square metal baking pan that is coated with cooking spray, and leave to bake for 20 minutes.
5. Next place cottage cheese in a food processor for 2 minutes or until smooth. Add granulated sugar, all-purpose flour, fresh lemon juice, grated lemon rind, baking sugar and egg (through egg white) and bend. Pour mixture over crust.
6. Let to bake at 350 degrees F. for 25 minutes or until the edges turn light brown. When cool, cover and refrigerated for 8 hours.
7. WHEN IT'S TIME TO SERVE, SPRINKLE WITH POWDERED SUGAR IF YOU DESIRE.

Dandelion-Stuffed Pork Loin

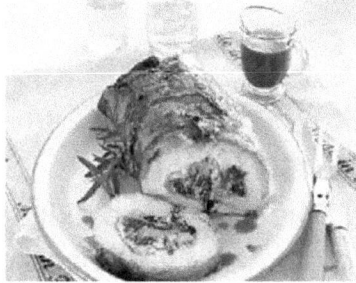

What you will need
Pork:
2 tablespoons olive oil
2 tablespoons chopped fresh rosemary
8 garlic cloves, minced
1/2 cup pitted dates, chopped
1/2 cup chopped onion
1/2 cup muscardine wine or any other sweet white wine
Cooking spray
1/4 pound thinly sliced pancetta
3/4 teaspoon kosher
1 cup panko (Japanese breadcrumbs)
1 boneless pork loin roast, trimmed
1/4 cup raisins, soaked in 1 cup water
3 (7-ounce) bunches dandelion greens, trimmed
Sauce:
2 1/2 tablespoons cornstarch
2 teaspoons butter

1/4 cup any dry white wine
1 cup fat-free, lower-sodium chicken broth
1/4 any sweet white wine
1 teaspoon water

How to prepare
1. Preheat oven to 450 degrees F.
2. Preparing pork, heat a large skillet over medium heat, and oil to pan. Add garlic and onion; sauté for 3 minutes. Next, add greens, 1/2 cup muscardine, pitted dates, raisins and cook until greens wilt, about 4 minutes (ensure it is covered).
3. Uncover and cook for an additional 3 minutes or until liquid evaporates.
4. Pulse greens mixture 3 times in a food processor, and then transfer to a bowl. Add rosemary, breadcrumbs, and 1/4 teaspoon salt. Toss to combine.
5. Cut pork through the center with a knife and open flat like a book. Place pork between 2 sheets of plastic wrap and pound with small heavy skillet to an even thickness.
6. Spread pancetta and dandelion over pork, allowing a 1/2-inch margin around outside edges. Next, roll up pork, jelly-roll fashion, starting with the short side.
7. Place pork in a shallow pan that's coated with cooking spray, and let to bake at 450 degrees for 15 minutes. Reduce oven temperature to 325 degrees and bake an additional 300 minutes, or until a

thermometer dipped in center reads 145 degrees. Transfer pork to a tray, reserving drippings n pa. Cover pork and let stand for 10 minutes.

8. Preparing sauce, stir 1/4 cup muscadine, broth, and white wine into pan drippings. Then pour wine mixture in a small saucepan. In a small bowl, mix 1 tablespoon water and cornstarch. Add the mixture to broth mixture and cook 1 minute, constantly stirring.

9. PUT DOWN FROM HEAT AND STIR IN BUTTER. CUT PORK INTO 14 SLICES (OR HOW YOU WISH), AND SERVE WITH SAUCE.

Cranberry Rolls

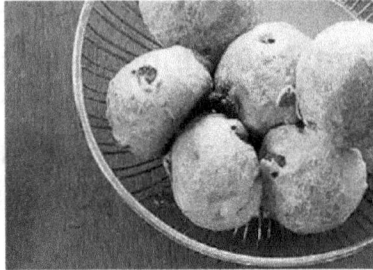

With a total time of 4o minutes, this recipe will yield 24 spicy rolls. Very low in sodium; you can be rest assured your low salt target isn't compromised.

What you will need
1/3 cup sugar
1/4 teaspoon salt
1 cup half-and-half
4 cups all-purpose flour
1 1/2 teaspoon ground ginger
1 teaspoon ground nutmeg
2 large eggs, beaten
1 teaspoon ground allspice
1 1/4 teaspoon cinnamon
2 1/4-oz. packets rapid-rise yeast
5 ½ tablespoons unsalted butter, cut into pieces
1 cup chopped fresh cranberries

How to prepare

1. Over medium heat, stir half-and-half sat, sugar, and 4 tbsp butter in a pan until thermometer reads 125 F.
2. Mix yeast, flour, and spices in a bowl. Toss in cranberries, stir in eggs and half-and-half mixture, until a ball forms
3. Turn dough out on a floured surface and knead for 6 minutes or until smooth. Cover for 9 minutes. Then line 2 baking sheets with parchment, coated with cooking spray.
4. Cut dough into 24 pieces; shape them into balls and place on sheets. Cover and let for 30 minutes to rise.
5. Preheat oven to 400 degrees F. Next, melt remaining 1 1/2 tbsp butter, brush onto the rolls and leave to bake for 18 minutes, or until golden brown.
6. ENSURE TO SWITCH THE SHEETS HALFWAY THROUGH. TAP A ROLL ON THE BOTTOM; IF IT SOUNDS HOLLOW, TURN OFF OVEN AND ALLOW ROLLS TO COOL. SERVE WARM.

Blueberry and Yogurt Soup with Lime swirl

Attractive, tasty and quick low-sodium side dish for lunch; you really have nothing to lose. When served with about 1 1/4, it will yield 4 servings.

What you will need
1/2 cup honey
Juice and zest of 1 medium lime
1/2 teaspoon cinnamon
1 1/2 teaspoons sugar
2 tablespoons plus 1 1/2 cups plain Greek yogurt (not nonfat)
4 cups blueberries

How to prepare
1. Keep some blueberries for garnish. Place remaining blueberries in a saucepan and add 1/2 cup water. Stir in cinnamon and honey and bring to simmer over medium-high heat, about 6 minutes.
2. Cook, stirring occasionally, until berries soften, about 3 minutes. Afterwards, transfer to a bowl and leave to cool slightly.
3. Smoothly blend blueberry mixture in a blender, and then transfer to a large bowl. Cover and let to refrigerate for 2 hours at least.
4. Mix lime juice, 2 tbsp yogurt, sugar, and lime zest in a small bowl, and stir to blend. Cover and refrigerate until soup is ready to be served.

5. Before serving, whisk remaining cup yogurt into blueberry mixture. Ladle soup into chilled bowls and pour 2 teaspoon of lime-yogurt mixture into center of each bowl.

6. MAKE DECORATIVE SWIRLS USING THE TIP OF A SHARP KNIFE, GARNISH WITH RESERVED BLUEBERRIES AND SERVE CHILLED.

Grilled Basil Chicken and Tomatoes

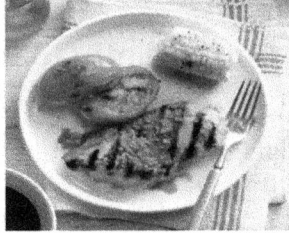

Delicious side dish with very little sodium content. In case you do not want salt at all ignore adding 1/4 teaspoon salt in the dish.

Total time: 25 minutes

Servings: 4

Nutritional facts: 1 serving; 5g fat, 8g carbohydrate, 24g protein, 177 calories, 98mg sodium

What you will need

4 boneless, skinless chicken breast halves (4 ounces each)

8 plum tomatoes

2 garlic gloves, minced

3/4 balsamic vinegar

2 tablespoons olive oil

1/4 teaspoon salt

1/4 cup tightly packed fresh basil leaves

How to prepare

1. Place the first five ingredients in a blender and cut 4 tomatoes into quarters.

2. Add to blende; cover and blend until smooth. Ensure to halve remaining tomatoes for grilling.
3. Combine chicken and 2/3 cup marinade in a bowl; refrigerate, covered, about 1 hour, stirring occasionally
4. Reserve the remaining marinade until it's time to serve.
5. Over medium heat, place chicken on an oiled grill rack and discard marinade remaining in the bowl.
6. Grill chicken for 4-6 minutes per side. Then grill tomatoes over medium heat until lightly browned, about 2-4 minutes per side.
7. SERVE THE CHICKEN AND TOMATOES WITH REMAINING MARINADE.

Low sodium recipes

Heart Healthy Muffins

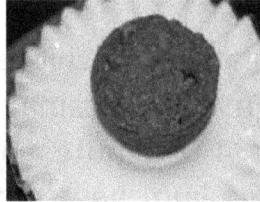

INGREDIENTS

- 3/4 cup unbleached flour
- 3/4 cup whole wheat pastry flour
- 3/4 cup oat bran
- 3/4 cup flax seed meal
- 1 cup brown sugar
- 2 teaspoons baking soda
- 1 teaspoon baking powder
- 1/2 teaspoon salt (optional)
- 2 teaspoons cinnamon
- 1 1/2 cups carrots, shredded
- 2 apples, peeled & shredded
- 1/2 cup raisins (optional)
- 1 cup nuts, chopped
- 3/4 cup soymilk
- 2 eggs, beaten
- 1 teaspoon vanilla

DIRECTIONS

- First of all combine and together flour flaxseed meal oat bran cook sugar hot soda fair powder nutrition if true and cinnamon into a large bowl add in carrots apples raisins if lust and nuts mixture milk hammer eggs and vanilla pour liquid ingredients and together into dry ingredients add till ingredients are moistened do not outer combine fill muffin cups 2/3 full.

Heart Healthy Cornbread

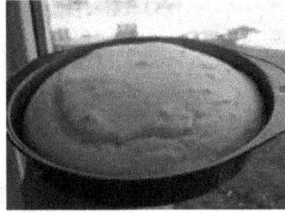

INGREDIENTS

- 1 cup cornmeal (I used half polenta half cornmeal)
- 1 cup unbleached flour (can use whole grain also)
- 1/4 cup oil
- 1 cup skim milk
- 2 egg whites (I used 1 whole egg)
- 1 tablespoon sugar (that plenty for me, but if desired use up to 4 tabs)
- 3 teaspoons baking powder
- 1/2 cup corn kernel (fresh or canned or thawed) (optional)

DIRECTIONS

- First of all mixture flour cornmeal hot powder hint if using see type and sugar in a big bowl in a second bowl beat together egg whites or egg milk and oil add into dry ingredients and together till just mixture add in corn nubbin if using and load into sauce tin either a 7 inch pie plate or muffin tins preheat at 380°F just for 18 minutes till tester comes out clean enjoy.

Cereal Heart Healthy

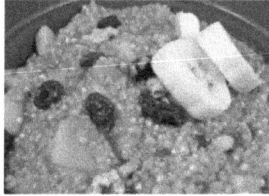

INGREDIENTS

- 1/2 cup steel cut oats
- 1/2 cup quinoa (well rinsed)
- 1 apple, cored and coarsely chopped (unpeeled)
- 1 teaspoon cinnamon
- 2 tablespoons raisins or 2 tablespoons dried blueberries, and or 2 tablespoons dried cranberries
- 2 tablespoons walnuts, toasted and rough chopped
- 2 cups water

TOPPINGS

- Raw honey
- Banana, sliced (optional)
- Berries (optional)

DIRECTIONS

- First of all steel cut oats quinoa cored and coarsely fell combine first three ingredients and together only for the toppings in a pot and sell to a boil decrease heat and boil coated for about 19 to 29 minutes rely on size and juiciness of the apple you may poverty more liquid adjust therefore by adding water or juice add and treat with raw fawn banana and rice milk.

Heart Healthy Smoothie

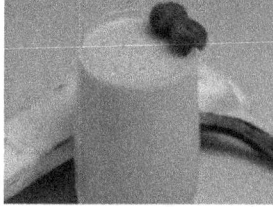

INGREDIENTS

- 1 (6 ounce) cartons your favorite yogurt
- 1 bananas or 1 fruit
- 1/3 cup cranberry-raspberry juice
- 1 tablespoon soy powder
- 1/2 cup crushed ice (MORE ICE if you want it thicker)

DIRECTIONS

- First of all stir ice to food processor with juice stir stay ingredients and together cutter till stocky enjoy.

www.ingramcontent.com/pod-product-compliance
Lightning Source LLC
Chambersburg PA
CBHW062133020426
42335CB00013B/1206